Leaky Bodies and Boundaries

D0165678

Drawing on postmodernist analyses, *Leaky Bodies and Boundaries* presents a feminist investigation into the marginalisation of women within a western discourse that denies both female moral agency and embodiment. With reference to contemporary and historical issues in biomedicine, the book argues that neither the boundaries of the subject nor the body are secure. The aim is both to valorise women and to suggest that 'leakiness' may be the very ground for a postmodern feminist ethic.

The book considers the biomedical body, both in relation to images from the early modern period, and to new reproductive technologies. Just as those bodies 'leak', so too does the structure of sameness and difference that shapes the modernist epistemology, ontology and ethics from which the parameters of bioethics derive. The enquiry – transdisciplinary throughout – is strongly influenced by the discursive approach of both Foucault and Derrida, but their indifference to feminist concerns is qualified in the light of strategies developed by Irigaray and Spivak, among others. Most importantly, *Leaky Bodies and Boundaries* goes on to reclaim sexual difference, in which the female is no longer the other of the male, and to draw from that an ethics of the body.

The contribution made by *Leaky Bodies and Boundaries* is to go beyond modernist feminisms – which simply add the female into existing paradigms – to radically displace and overflow the mechanisms by which women are devalued. The anxiety that postmodernism cannot yield an ethics, nor advance feminist concerns is also addressed.

Margrit Shildrick, formerly Convenor and Lecturer in Women's Studies at the University of Leeds, is now an Honorary Research Fellow at the University of Liverpool.

Leaky Bodies and Boundaries

Feminism, postmodernism and (bio)ethics

Margrit Shildrick

London and New York

HQ
1190
.S43
1997

First published 1997
by Routledge
11 New Fetter Lane, London EC4P 4EE

Simultaneously published in the USA and Canada
by Routledge
29 West 35th Street, New York, NY 10001

© 1997 Margrit Shildrick

Typeset in Times by Florencetype Ltd, Stoodleigh, Devon

Printed and bound in Great Britain by Biddles Ltd, Guildford and
King's Lynn

All rights reserved. No part of this book may be reprinted or
reproduced or utilized in any form or by any electronic,
mechanical, or other means, now known or hereafter
invented, including photocopying and recording, or in any
information storage or retrieval system, without permission in
writing from the publishers.

British Library Cataloguing in Publication Data
A catalogue record for this book is available from the British Library

Library of Congress Cataloging in Publication Data
A catalogue record for this book has been requested

ISBN   0–415–14616–X
       0–415–14617–8 (pbk)

LONGWOOD COLLEGE LIBRARY
FARMVILLE, VIRGINIA 23901

Contents

LONGWOOD LIBRARY
1000298090

List of illustrations

Figures 1.1 and 1.3–1.9 are reproduced courtesy of the Wellcome
Institute Library, London; figure 1.2 courtesy of Serono Ltd; figure
1.10 courtesy of the Benefits Agency

Acknowledgements

My thanks are due to all those who have contributed time and energy towards the completion of this book. Most particularly, I am endebted to Christine Battersby, Hilary Graham, Janet Price and Catherine Constable, who have between them provided the stimulus of an unflagging and meticulous critique, multiple rereadings, feminist insight, inspiration and encouragement. At a more distant level, the responses to the original manuscript given by Joanna Hodge, Selma Sevenhuijsen and Ros Diprose have stimulated some important clarifications. And throughout the project both Lis Davidson and Liz MacGarvey have offered no less important and sustaining support at many other levels.

I am grateful to Michele Minto of the Wellcome Iconographic Library, at the Wellcome Institute for the History of Medicine, London, for help in tracing many of the pre-nineteenth-century images referred to in the first part of Chapter 1.

The section of Chapter 1 which deals with anatomy and representation forms the basis of a joint illustrated presentation given at the 1993 Women's Studies Network (UK) Conference, and subsequently published as 'Splitting the difference' (Shildrick and Price 1994). Parts of Chapter 2 draw on work previously published as 'Women, bodies and consent' (Shildrick 1992); and in Chapter 6, the section entitled 'Mis(sed)conceptions' has appeared in the *Journal of Medicine and Philosophy*, vol. 22, 1997.

Introduction

[L]aughter in the face of serious categories is indispensable for feminism.

(Butler 1990, *Gender Trouble*)

The theme of this book is women, bodies and ethics and the way in which all of those might be recuperated within postmodernism. In view of the latter's reputation for chaotic free-fall, for indifference to the ethical, and for a hostility to both gender categories and to the material, the task is a not inconsiderable one. In breaching boundaries, as I intend to do, I am nonetheless constrained to proceed with due gravity and caution. But postmodern scepticism is both weighty and playful, and the feminism I endorse is finally a celebratory one.

As an historically important subdivision of philosophy, the study of ethics – that is, the principles governing moral being and moral behaviour – has produced numerous more or less monolithic systems of explanation. The task of meta-ethics and of normative ethics, both of which operate from a position of supposed detachment, has been respectively to clarify and comment upon the meaning of the operative terms – the good, right, justice, and so on – and to compare and order competing systems. And the further goal of substantive ethics is to insert into practice whichever theoretical principles are privileged. Application may be directed towards promoting those character traits which constitute being moral in oneself, as in the tradition of Aristotelianism and recent virtue ethics, or it may focus on promoting particular forms of behaviour as constitutive of morality, as variously adduced by the principles of deontology or consequentialism, for example.

To all these areas feminism has over the last few years turned its critical gaze, not least because of the growing realisation that women, in Western societies at least,[1] have been ill-served by the tenets of existing systems. What is at issue is not simply that morality seems largely to be about and for men – what kind of man should the moral person be? how should a man act morally towards others? – but that its very terms and conditions are constructed in such a way as inherently to exclude women from consideration. The marginalisation of women is not confined simply to the material organisation of socio-political structures, like medicine and the law, but is evident in the very foundation of the Western logos, in the processes of reasoning and articulation through which meaning is produced. This is no small charge, for what follows is the need to question not just ethics but epistemology and ontology as well. If the feminist project, within which I situate my own work, is about valorising women, about re-visioning our being in the world, then a feminist-inspired ethic must do more than simply extend the scope of morality. The exposure and critique of the fallacious claims to gender neutrality in which conventional ethics has clothed itself is a necessary step, but what also becomes apparent is that the justificatory appeal to universalism, and the illusion of objectivity and impartiality on which that is based, is unlikely to be sustainable. And in so far as Western ethics has based itself not simply on the exclusion of women as moral agents, but makes transcendent disembodiment a condition of agency, then a new approach will insist on re-inscribing the bodies of women.

The postmodernist perspective, which I shall with reservations employ, is a problematic one for feminism precisely because it seems to undermine not only the hitherto entrenched givens of a male en-gendered epistemology, but also the very ground on which women might seek to position their own project. In so far as the deconstruction of boundaries and the recognition of radical differences is at the heart of postmodernist feminist enterprise, the very category of 'women' becomes difficult to appeal to in any unambiguous way. Where signification is acknowledged as slippery and treacherous, the issue becomes not the creation of new normative standards, but a persistent endeavour to forefront the instability and provisionality[2] of the concepts with which one is dealing. This will be addressed in greater depth later in the text, but for the moment what needs to be marked is that the understanding and prospective application of the alternative ethic which I shall propose as more appropriate to feminist critique cannot aim at closure. There is no final absolute answer to moral dilemmas, no self-complete system which can satisfy all the demands made of it, nor which can speak with authority across time and place. I am not even sure that it should seek to depose existing systems in the sense of making them entirely redundant, but should rather contextualise and limit the grounds of their applications. The point is that a feminist ethic asks different questions of itself. It seeks to understand the specificity of meanings and the particularity of participants, with the result that its answers must always be held open to modification at least, and possibly to radical change. In the same way the 'ethic' itself, as a theoretical construct, builds in its own provisionality, its own rejection of certainty, and accordingly it makes no universal claims. Yet that very openness is often taken by detractors as the mark of the impossibility of forming any postmodernist projects. It is, nonetheless, fully cognisant with one strand of feminist theorising, and in that context can be recuperated, I believe, to serve our ends as women. Openness should not be interpreted as weakness, nor as indecision, but rather as the courage to refuse the comforting refuge of broad categories and fixed unidirectional vision.

The conduct of philosophy in the West has been ill prepared to accept any form of feminist challenge to it, save perhaps the call for reformist adjustments which leave the basis of the canon untouched. I shall mention here two major strands of that canon, dominant since the Enlightenment. First, despite a history of enquiry into the reliability of what Locke, in *An Essay Concerning Human Understanding*, calls 'sensation' and 'reflection' (1975, Book 2), there is a common-sense assumption that objectivity is possible. In other words, there are pre-existing facts – with regard both to external nature and to ourselves – which we are able to access unmediated by preconceptions or values. Moreover, language is simply the transparent vehicle of pre-given meaning. As Elizabeth Grosz remarks: 'the ideal of a truth that presents itself directly to consciousness in "pure" form, without the mediation of anything extraneous haunts western knowledges' (1990: 93). The second strand holds that in the exercise of reason we are guaranteed progress toward the elimination of evils and the final emancipation of human beings. It is nonetheless a philosophy of boundaries and exclusions, and one that has not proved adequate to the aspirations of women. Recently, however, the self-critique generated from within modernist philosophy has provided the opportunity for more radical feminisms to contest those exclusions which have displaced or effaced the feminine voice. But allowing that gender awareness has been a relatively late addition to philosophical theorisation, it is by no means clear, despite the best attempts to write in the feminine, that the valorisation of real women has been or can be secured. From the most reformist liberal feminism which seeks simply to realise the promise of equality, to the most pointed critical theory with its stress on the emancipation of the subject, the impact of feminist theory has been blunted, I would maintain, by the failure to question either the foundational claims of philosophy or the status not just of the female subject, but of any subject.

Although I shall allude constantly to such feminisms, my analysis is directed elsewhere, and most particularly towards the possibilities of a feminist take-up of poststructuralism and postmodernism. Indeed, my contention is that it is only that approach which can provide feminism with the tools sufficient to disrupt masculinist philosophy radically and to make a place for a reconceived feminine. In order to be valorised *as* women, we have a stake in recuperating some form of sexual specificity, and what a postmodernist feminism may empower is a feminine that is excessive to the closure of binary sexual difference. What poststructuralism has done is to begin to prise open the cracks, to expose those gaps and silences that undermine the claims of modernist philosophy to impartiality and universality. Above all, it deconstructs the boundaries between categories, be they ontological, epistemological, ethical or material; and it demonstrates the inescapability of the leaks and flows across all such bodies of knowledge and bodies of matter. Recent feminist theory has appropriated the methodologies of postmodernism to occupy the newly opened spaces, to exploit the fluidity between margins and centre, not so much with gratitude as with the determination to critique not just the conventions of modernity, but, in many cases, the male progenitors and masculinist uses of postmodernism itself. Nonetheless, the turn to postmodernism, as I shall discuss, entails ambiguities and risks for the feminist project, and it is as necessary to avoid the reification of the postmodern as it is the violent foreclosures of modernism.

Given that the valorisation of women remains a central aim of feminism, the new orthodoxies may be as suspect as their predecessors. And for all its dispersal of rigid categories there is a sense in which postmodernist *philosophy*, with its sometimes slavish concentration on the text, still excludes from consideration the kind of interdisciplinary approach now considered intrinsic to feminist enquiry. I prefer Deleuze's idea of 'deterritorialisation', and make no apology then for an approach which consciously crosses boundaries and makes use of insights from a variety of disciplines. Nor do I claim that every author I cite in support of my own analysis would consistently hold that particular point of view, still less approve the use to which I may put it. My point is not that scholarship should be decontextualised and treated as free-floating; on the contrary, feminist thinking is marked, characteristically, by an acknowledgement of its own situatedness and its partiality in terms of both bias and lack of completion. What matters is that ways of knowing should be dynamic, and indeed the static authorial relationship between writer, text and reader is one which it is the business of postmodernism to contest. Though I shall both build on and deconstruct the familiar material of ethics, I hope that my conclusions will move beyond it to construct an understanding that no longer relies on the inadequate analyses of one particular perspective. My method is that of the *bricoleur*,[3] not of the academic philosopher, and perhaps a properly based enterprise in women's studies demands no less.

For the purposes of my argument, poststructuralism and postmodernism may be treated in some respects as synonymous, especially in so far as each constitutes a critique of modernity, and most particularly of its liberal humanist form. By liberal humanism I mean that conception of the moral and social order, dominant since the seventeenth-century Enlightenment, in which gender-neutral, individual and autonomous actors conduct their own lives and enter into contractual relations with other individuals on the basis of free will and rationality. Now, strictly speaking, poststructuralism encompasses a set of theories characterised by rigorous anti-humanism and anti-subjectivity, and by the claim that all knowledge is discursively constructed. The term 'postmodernism' has, in comparison, a more extended use outside the linguistic and philosophical context, and has come to denote a range of cultural theories and practices which break with the unity and certainty of the Western intellectual tradition. For my purposes, however, I take postmodernism to devolve on the following considerations:

1 the rational/scientific project of the Enlightenment has ended, with the consequent fragmentation of a coherent notion of truth and knowledge into a series of dispersed, competing and conflicting discourses;
2 because appeal to a unified rationality or morality is no longer plausible, the teleological ideals of the 'grand narratives' of liberal humanism, science (including medical discourse), the law, and so on must be abandoned;
3 the human subject is just one such ideal configuration and as such can no longer individually authorise knowledge claims; and the notion of subjectivity itself is deeply problematised;
4 the boundaries between hitherto discrete bodies of knowledge have blurred to challenge both the hierarchical organisation of distinct disciplines and the division between theory and practice.

Although these criteria would seem to imply – and many cultural critics would claim – that our own age is indeed postmodern, I would argue that there is no necessary coincidence between post-modernity and any specific historical epoch. The analysis I use can be, and is, directed at uncovering the inherent instabilities in all discourses, and moreover, its aim is not to falsify past claims so much as to disrupt them. The certainty of categorical distinctions may be shattered, but deconstruction is not synonymous with destruction, and we are entitled to recuperate some elements and look for new – albeit provisional – configurations of meaning and value.

The area of traditional ethics from which I shall launch my critique is that of moral agency, by which is meant the sense in which an individual can be said to be in control of and responsible for choices made and acted on within the moral sphere. Yet what I shall move on to is not so much a feminist reconstruction of general principles or rules of behaviour, as an ethic in which differences are acknowledged, respected and allowed to flourish as the very basis of moral discourse. And the embodiment of those differences, rather than their abstraction, will be taken as a determining feature of a specifically feminist approach. I shall look in particular at how traditional notions are applied within bio-medicine, using that term, as do Beauchamp and Childress (1983), as a shorthand expression for the interactive field of science, medicine and health care. It is a field where the technological developments of the late twentieth century have placed especial strain on conventional ethical paradigms. The nexus of procedures collectively referred to as New Reproductive Technologies (hereafter NRTs[4]), including some which, like artificial insemination, are neither new nor technically sophisticated, provides one area in which that strain is clearly exemplified. In so far as many biomedical technologies now in use, or anticipated, exhibit at least some of the features listed above, I shall assume that they are consistent with what is understood as postmodern, and as such may highlight the challenge to traditional conceptions of bioethics. Given the central concern with the bodies and well-being of women, NRTs have become a focus for feminist enquiry, which has in turn generated competing accounts of how we may best address the problems and demands of the postmodern world. It has not always been clear, or at least it has rarely been explicit, that biomedicine should be subject to moral scrutiny, and it is perhaps around the issues arising from areas such as that of NRTs that it has become increasingly recognised that all forms of intervention in human lives have ethical implications.

The last few decades have seen, in the Anglo-American context at least, a marked expansion of ethical interest in health-care issues, and the spawning of a distinct discipline generally termed 'medical ethics' or 'bioethics'. A proliferation of texts has appeared which go well beyond the fixed certainties of the past and posit a problematic in which the health-care encounter is seen as one which must be negotiated with as much ethical as technical acuity. It is not that the transactions of health care have entirely escaped moral scrutiny in the past,[5] but that the issue was assumed to rest on the proper conduct of the practitioner. So long as she[6] was seen to be exercising appropriate moral agency, according to parameters already laid down within implicit and explicit professional codes, then the moral requirement was satisfied. The position of the other participant – the patient – in the health-care encounter was of limited ethical interest in that she was characterised as a passive receiver of benefits rather than as an independent agent. The dichotomy between the two positions, that of the morally active professional and of the inactive patient, was most clearly evidenced in the traditional medical model of health care in which the two roles were clearly delineated on an institutional level. Though it most often centres on the narrower limits of medicine rather than on health care as a whole, modern ethical scrutiny – and I mean here, of course, ethics in its humanist context – has opened up the encounter to an analysis which increasingly insists on the moral positioning of *both* participants. Whereas for some the emphasis remains on the discharge of professional duties, in the context of which the patient's part is satisfied by some notion of concomitant rights, more radical analyses seek to extend full moral agency itself to the patient as participant.

In such an ideal scenario, then, the medical encounter would become not simply an intervention on the part of an active participant into the life of a passive one, but a transaction between two self-determining moral agents. Indeed, self-determination may stand as the perceived *sine qua non* of moral agency and hence for moral discourse, but it is nevertheless evident that its manifestation in practice is severely restricted. The question arises as to whether it is possible to reconcile theory and practice on existing models, or does the very gap between real and ideal suggest that the notion of mutual moral agency is incompatible both with traditional models of health care and with the structuration of ethical paradigms? I shall suggest that the deconstruction of the apparently gender-neutral terms of the problematic will make clear not only the inherent implausibility of establishing the humanist ideal in terms of the medical model, but will also contest a philosophical tradition which places autonomy at the centre of moral agency. By employing a specifically postmodernist feminist perspective, however, it is not simply the parameters of moral agency that are called into question, but the very possibility of ethics itself.

While both the deconstruction of the gender binaries which have served to ground the discursive and material oppression of the category of women, and the deconstruction of the closure of prior and exclusionary models of knowledge, are clearly to be welcomed, what generates a widespread feminist resistance to postmodernism is precisely its apparent inability to deliver any political or ethical agenda. There is undeniably a problem in that the poststructuralist problematisation of all standards, regardless of their perceived value, and the associated denial of concepts such as progress, stable subjectivity and the immediacy of the real do seem to undercut fatally any programme directed towards a better life. The difficulty is exacerbated moreover in the tendency of postmodernism to operate at a highly abstract level where there is little place for an understanding of substantive issues, such as those which constitute the practices of biomedicine, for example. Feminist theory cannot undertake to resolve these issues fully, but neither need it turn its back on what I take to be the most radical opportunity of shaking off a legacy that has failed women – indeed all those who are 'others' – and entering instead into alternative modes of being, knowing and acting.

What I am concerned to outline in this work are the conditions for the possibility of an ethics; to ask what emerges when identity and difference are no longer the ground on which moral discourse is constructed. In place of either effacing the oppositional difference in a move to sameness, or responding to the other as alien, a postmodernist approach uncovers both the *multiple* differences and distinctions that mediate interactions, and paradoxically the way in which all boundaries are permeable and ultimately indistinct. There are two things which mark my account as a specifically feminist take-up of postmodernism. First, though I consistently identify and critique the moves of sameness and difference which ground the liberal humanist project, I privilege an Irigarayan reading which *anticipates* a distinction between women and men.[7] As will become clearer as my argument emerges, what that entails is the recovery/discovery of a radical sexual difference, a difference that speaks to the feminine *beyond* the oppositional gender binary. Clearly, such an approach can answer to the demands for a female specificity, and, moreover, I believe it is consistent with a poststructuralist agenda. In evading the risk of moving from the deconstruction of the binary to a re-enacted gender indifference, what is being (re)claimed is not a homogeneous category of women, but rather a multiplicity of fluid positions linked only by the in-common experience of a specific body form. And that notion speaks precisely to my second feminist marker: the insistence that discursive deconstruction should not entail dis-embodiment.

Given that the devaluation of corporeality, or at very least ambivalence towards the body, has been a dominant feature of masculinist knowledge, my contention is that a resistant feminism must seek to explore the body anew. I shall argue that both the material body and the female are positioned as other to the transcendent subject and denied expression in ethical paradigms. And where the lived body *is* acknowledged as the site of subjectivity, as in phenomenology, it is nonetheless as a universalised masculine body. Moreover, that body is curiously absent to us during health, and it is only in sickness that it makes itself fully felt, and then as that which unsettles the sense of self. Effectively, neither the feminine nor the body itself are valorised as lived presences. In mainstream discourse, that devaluation is even more evident, and the denial more entrenched. Yet, at the same time, as a postmodernist analysis contends, the feminine and the body are each both absent and excessive. In other words, the boundaries of exclusion are never wholly secure against the threat of the absent other to disrupt the unity and definition of the selfsame. Indeed, the whole issue of inside/outside is one that this work will problematise, and with it, finally, the very sense that any body can be read as a discrete entity. Where the feminist agenda somewhat shifts the parameters of postmodernist enquiry, however, is in the refusal to read the body only as text. It is both the surface of inscription and the site of material practices, each of which speaks to a sexed specificity. Although intending to deconstruct the essentialism of the highly damaging historical elision between women and their bodies, postmodernist feminists might see, nevertheless, the embodiment of the feminine as precisely the site from which new forms of knowledge could emerge.[8]

In choosing to make bioethics the particular focus of my enquiry, I have intended to address head on the especial consequences of regarding the body itself as leaky. Once 'real' material entities as well as linguistic concepts are understood to be discursive constructions, then the practices of medicine and health care must necessarily be seen in a different light. It is not just that the concepts around the body, such as notions of health and disease, able-bodied and disabled, and so on, become problematic, but that biomedicine may be concerned as much with constituting the body as with restoring it. Yet despite a substantial literature on the construction of medical knowledge, there has been an almost complete silence within the field of health-care studies, of whatever discipline, on the significance of that further postmodernist insight. Notwithstanding some previous engagement with postmodernism, Sarah Nettleton, for example, makes little attempt to address the issues in her recent book *The Sociology of Health and Illness* (1995), while Deborah Lupton (1994, 1995) consistently cites a range of pertinent authors, but fails to develop fully and explore the implications of a critical approach. More relevant are the texts by Nicholas Fox (1993) and, more tangentially, by Ros Diprose (1994), which share my own approach in drawing on both Derridean *différance* and Foucault's understanding of embodiment, though there the similarities end. Where Fox merely gestures towards feminist theory and privileges a quasi-Deleuzean Body-without-Organs as the inscribed surface of medical discourse, Diprose evinces a characteristically feminist concern with the limitations and possibilities of a corporeal ethics. As I understand it, what is at stake in traditional health-care practices is that the material boundaries of the body should be secure and that otherness be excluded. Against that tradition, my own use of the concept of *différance*, like that of Diprose, serves to underline the ultimate instability of the biomedical task, and to claim that if bodies are not fixed, then nor are ethical relationships. Moreover, I am fully committed to the recuperation of embodied sexual difference as the certain co-instance of an ethic of intimate *and* irreducible differences.

My project starts and finishes then with bodies. Chapter 1 sets out the substantive underpinnings of bioethics and places the body in context as a discursive construct. In the first half I look at the historical construction of male and female bodies, and trace not the progressive acquisition of supposedly factual knowledge, but rather a series of ruptures organised around fluctuating paradigms of sameness and difference. The second part of the chapter moves on to apply – with reference to (dis)ability in particular – a broadly Foucauldian analysis to discern the imposition of disciplinary regimes, including that of biomedicine, to secure the material and corporeal within a stable and controllable framework. Chapter 2 outlines those systems of ethics dominant since the Enlightenment and looks at how their abstract tenets have been taken up within bioethics, and most particularly in the injunction to respect autonomy. The hidden gender assumptions of those general ethical and epistemological paradigms are investigated in some detail in the following chapter. I launch there a critique of modernity, and introduce poststructuralist theory as that which points up the fractures in those boundaries of certainty which marginalise and exclude the feminine. Chapter 4 discusses one conventional feminist perspective on ethics which associates an ethic of caring, and an attention to diversity, with a reformed liberal humanism. I then move on to consider some feminist responses to the difficulties posed by a more postmodernist approach. Chapter 5 picks up the issue at the centre of much feminist hostility to postmodernism and argues that the deconstruction of subjectivity results not in the dead-end of permanent fragmentation, but in the opening up of multiple possibilities for agency. Moreover, the emergence of sexual difference, in its Irigarayan sense of the difference that exceeds the binary, is consequent not least on the deconstruction of (male) presence. The chapter concludes with a discussion of the body and the phenomenological subject of health care, and argues that an ethic of difference must be embodied. That theme is taken up in specific detail in the final chapter which investigates the implications of the postmodern body for feminism, particularly as it is manifest in reproductive technologies. The transgressions effected by NRTs are the source of much ontological anxiety, but I suggest that their problematisation of the essentialist boundaries and of simple difference may be turned to feminist ends. In conclusion I offer a summary of what I have called the ethical moment which must precede ethics as such, and I recommend instability, multiplicity, the incalculable, and above all leakiness as the very ground for a postmodernist feminist ethic.

Chapter 1

Fabrica(tions)
On the construction of the human body

THE BIOMEDICAL BODY

To say that the human body is the focus of health care is an observation so obvious as to seem trivial, and yet in its unproblematised
form it is one major axis of the inadequacy of traditional health-
care ethics. In the convention, the ideal body of biomedicine is
taken to precede the operation of a bioethics which claims to offer
a moral analysis of the practices of the body. What I shall argue
in this chapter is that the body, as we know it, is a fabrication,
organised not according to an historically progressive discovery
of the real, but as an always insecure and inconsistent artefact,
which merely mimics material fixity. It is not, then, that a single
and unified discursive construct stands in for the givenness of the
real, but rather that a plethora of competing discourses resist any
final closure on the question of the body. With that in mind, I
have intentionally avoided a narrative structure to my exposition,
preferring instead to uncover an array of discontinuous and
discrete 'truths', associated one with the other only by a logic of
phallocentrism. The point is that for all their fluidity, not all
discourses are of equal status, and what I want to demonstrate is
how certain forms achieve dominance through normalisation and
reiteration. Moreover, by looking at a linked series of dichotomies
which underlay the cultural history of the West, I shall argue that,
although the bodies of women have figured strongly throughout,
they have been habitually conceptualised and valued in a quite
different way from those of men.

The so-called medical model, which has dominated the traditional biosciences, speaks to a powerful split between mind and
body whereby the knowing subject is disembodied, detached from

corporeal raw material. In a specific take-up of Merleau-Ponty (1962), however, one currently fashionable strand in the philosophy of medicine addresses health in terms of the being-in-the-world of bodies; that is, the sense in which our phenomenological stability is intrinsically tied up with the unified presence of our bodies (Gadow 1980; Leder 1984, 1990; Schenck 1986; Young 1984, 1990). The phenomenological claim is that the 'broken' body of sickness has important consequences for our self-perception, such that the loss of a leg or a breast, for example, affects not simply corporeal integrity, but also the sense of who we are. Nonetheless, I want to suggest that for women there are already a variety of paradoxes in play that deeply problematise the notion of the unity of mind and body that the phenomenological model presupposes. Moreover, whatever forms the dominant representation has taken, the bodies of women, whether all too present or disconcertingly absent, have served to ground the devaluation of women by men. What I am proposing is that it is the body itself, in whatever physical form it is experienced, which positions women as both morally deficient and existentially disabled. Even the 'whole' body of phenomenology is intrinsically masculine, and women, by that token, are never in full existential health.

It is important to mark from the outset that I am concerned not with 'real' bodies, but with the various and seemingly contradictory cultural constructions of them. This is to go a great deal further than to say simply that the concept of bodies as marked, either positively or negatively, by health is a social, and indeed moral, artefact. My intention is to contest the authority and apparent certainty of the real, not in order to deny materiality, but to insist that there is never direct, unmediated access to some 'pure' corporeal state. Such an emphasis on the lack of foundational substance for the objects of perception is a central facet of poststructuralism. It may best be understood as the move from a belief in naturally existent material – which may be more or less accurately represented – to a position that the act of representation itself is the moment of materialisation. More specifically, against the modern belief that we can grasp the supposedly transparent reality of the natural world, and ultimately of our own natures, I am claiming that what is taken to be the neutral, biological body is itself an effect of language. As Gayatri Spivak puts it: 'There are thinkings of the systematicity of the body, there are

value codings of the body. The body, as such, cannot be thought'
(1989b: 149). In other words, the body is always a discursive
construction, marked by environmental process and by power, but
given to us only in our texts. In short, we could always know it,
and its biology, in a different way, as indeed a genealogy of the
body would show. The Renaissance anatomists, for example, who
saw the female reproductive organs as homologous to male genitalia,[1] were neither unobservant nor simply bad scientists. The
'truth' they expressed was the truth of their age. This relationship between cultural values and constructions of the body, as
part of what Foucault would call the power/knowledge regime, is
a symbiotic one. 'The exercise of power perpetually creates knowledge and, conversely, knowledge constantly induces effects of
power' (1980: 52). Though the dominant discourse may dictate
certain conceptions of the body, those privileged conceptions are
rarely acknowledged as such. What then appears to be reality in
turn justifies and perpetuates particular truth claims. And what
concerns me here is which truths are given to, and derived from,
the female body in a male social order. The task of historical
enquiry, what Foucault called genealogy, is 'to expose a body
totally imprinted by history and the process of history's destruction of the body' (1977b: 148).[2] This is no abstract question for,
although perception and knowledge *are* always mediated, and
bodies themselves are discursive formations, what is done as a
result of those truths has of course real material effects which
have direct bearing on our lives as women.

For the moment, however, I want to look at the unproblematised medical model which is marked by its supposed gender
neutrality. The implicit assumption is that the body is some kind
of stable and unchanging given, differentiated simply by its variable manifestation of the signs and symptoms of health or disease,
ability or disability, normality or abnormality. At its most
schematic, the medical model favours a professional scientific
approach in which a reductionist concentration on the pathology
of the body serves to dehumanise the 'patient' and reduce her to
the status of a malfunctioning machine. The paradigm of the
human body, which grounds such a model, relies on a reading of
the dualistic concept of mind and body developed by Descartes
during the seventeenth century. Although that particular form is
both less complex and more consistent than his further proposals
suggest, it is basic Cartesian dualism which has continued to

dominate popular, medical and philosophical views in the West for the succeeding 300 years. The model is, as always, culturally specific and never without contemporaneous counter-discourses, but it does nevertheless mark a paradigm shift in the concept of embodiment. In elaborating the so-called mind/body split in *A Discourse on Method* and other works, Descartes clearly intended that it should have medical application. Briefly, in a traditional reading, the Cartesian model ascribes to mind alone – the *res cogitans* – the powers of intelligence and animation, spirituality and selfhood, while the corporeal body – the *res extensa* – becomes simply a machine susceptible to a mathematical–causal analysis of functioning.

The concept of some kind of binary split between body and soul was not of course new to the early modern period. Arguably, it has been a dominant form since the inception of Christianity, which itself incorporated strands of Platonist dualism within its episteme. Nor does the corresponding relative devaluation of the body represent a radical change in itself. What does seem to be different, however, is the nature of that devaluation. Whereas, in Cartesian terms, the body is something to be rejected as an obstacle to pure rational being, in early Christian texts, the body was conceptualised as the necessary path to higher spirituality. The mortification of the present flesh, so vividly portrayed in medieval primers on the lives of the saints, for example,[3] was simply a stage on the way to the final recuperation of the perfectly embodied soul. The move to the notion of the body as (a machine) other than/of the self is a modern one which sanctions not so much that self-absorbed bodily fetishism as a spirit of disciplined objectification. And yet though the denial and devaluation of embodiment has been claimed as a characteristic feature of modernity, that negation remains nevertheless contradictory and precarious. While the practice of disciplinary power over one's own body or the bodies of others can evidence detachment, even indifference, it speaks too to a persisting anxiety posed by the threat of corporeal engulfment. Moreover, as a more specifically gendered analysis will show, the female sex stands in a different relationship to embodiment than does the male, such that women both exemplify the effect of, and manifest, that threat. What I have in mind is both the especial immanence of the female body, as it is frequently represented in ontological theory, such that it enmeshes women themselves; and its putative leakiness, the outflow of the body which breaches the boundaries of the proper.[4] Those differences – mind/body, self/other, inner/outer – which should remain clear and distinct are threatened by loss of definition, or by dissolution. And though that might be appropriated as a positive image of fluid boundaries, as some poststructuralist/postmodern feminists and notably Luce Irigaray have done, in the male cultural imaginary the metaphor characteristically provokes unease, even horror.[5] This is no less true in health care than elsewhere.

Without making any grand narrative claims of cause and effect, it is clear that a dualist construction of bodily being served well the development of a mechanistic medical science in which the corporeal body could be mapped, measured and experimented on without moral impediment. The technological and clinical advances, which emerged within the wider discursive environment of the early modern period, figured the self not only as extrinsic to the body, but the body as an essentially socially isolated, self-contained mechanism. As such, it could in effect be taken apart, both to see how it worked in its structural complexity and to rectify functional faults. The growing use of empirical methodology enabled physicians to isolate specific causes, and to theorise a construction both of disease and of the 'normal' body of health to which it was counterposed. The reductionism inherent in the empirical method became the very essence of the new medical model, which was set up as rational, unbiased, neutral and objective. As the concept of health was both established as a recognisable regulatory norm, and progressively narrowed to mean simply the absence of disease, the specialism of medicine became the dominant form of health care. At the same time, medicine expanded its remit as the potential location of disease was broadened to encompass such areas as that of sexuality or the emotions. Practitioners were increasingly seen as men of science, acting as skilled technicians, whose expert knowledge could lead to the elimination of the disease state wherever it might occur. On a formal level, then, the institution of modern medicine is firmly rooted in the idea that health is some kind of given: a normative state which can be restored by defeating the abnormality of disease.[6] Not surprisingly, this dualist model has clear implications for what kind of morality might be appropriate to the practice of medicine, and by extension to health care as a whole.

That the early modern emphasis was less on bodily integrity than on increasing differentiation of body parts is evidenced by the demand, both scientific and popular, for serial diagrams of human anatomy. What I have in mind, for instance, are the extraordinary and much imitated Vesalian drawings in the 'Epitome' of *De humani corporis fabrica* (1543) which show the body progressively stripped of its skin and muscle to reveal the underlying skeleton, or the so-called fugitive sheets popular in the seventeenth century whereby successive flaps are lifted to reveal the internal organs. Similar pedagogic aids persist into the twentieth century, and remain indicative of the cultural ideals of each particular society. What is the more remarkable in many of the early examples is that the physical body and the motivational self are so clearly assumed to be discontinuous that the 'person' appears to assist in his own dissection. A proudly upright figure may display his own flayed skin, pull aside his musculature the better to display deeper structures, or may point out her own internal organs (Figure 1.1).

And once the body has been constructed as ontologically and structurally differentiated in this way, then the division into discrete systems or parts grounds a reductive approach to medical practice. The task of the physician, conceived in the ideal as that of a wholly rational and objective scientist, is simply to cure the body and restore it to (functional) normality. Although there are contexts in which this may be a legitimate priority, the problem lies in making it a general condition. The essence of such health work is dispassionate intervention on the part of the professional into an essentially passive body. And though in practice that ideal may be compromised, there is, too, little sense in formal medical ethics that health care may involve mutual participation in a joint endeavour, or that, despite new constructions of the late modern body which privilege a unified systems approach, the integrity of the patient as person may be at stake. What is held to be appropriate in both legal and moral codes remains largely grounded on the medical model [7] whereby the body is simply the site of objective intervention into the disease

Figure 1.1   (a) Mundinus: *Anatomia* (1541). Female figure on parturition chair. Courtesy Wellcome Institute Library, London
(b) Juan Valverde de Hamusco: *Anatomia del corpo humano* (1560). Male figure. Courtesy Wellcome Institute Library, London

(a)

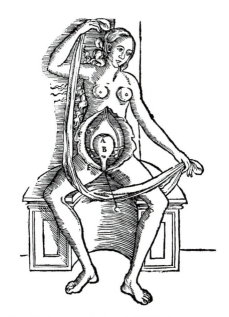

(b)

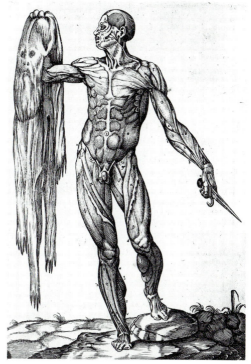

process, rather than the focus of a holistic concern with the person. As Foucault puts it in *The Birth of the Clinic,* 'one did not think first of the internal structure of the organised being, but of the medical bipolarity of the normal and the pathological' (1973: 35).

Nonetheless, as Foucault goes on to outline, historically 'medical thought is fully engaged with the philosophical status of man' (ibid.: 198). What characterises the pre-modern holistic model of the body was its construction as an abstract entity, marked by the humours or corresponding to the cosmos, for example, but known not individually, nor through singular observation, but through the guidance of authoritative texts. What, for Foucault, prepares the ground for the move to modern clinical medicine was a shift, during the sixteenth and seventeenth centuries, in the nature of post-mortem examination whereby speculative reason gave way to the science of observation. Nonetheless, as Laqueur (1990a) has outlined at some length, classical medical knowledge, itself dominated by Galen's dissections not of humans but of animals, remained influential long after the revival of anatomy and was not finally displaced for another 200 years. The traditional explanation for the centuries-long eclipse of human anatomy – a discipline which in any case may never have amounted to more than an *ad hoc* practice (Philips 1987) – and its disappearance from medical education after the early Classical period is rejected by Foucault. In his view, what had effected the change was not so much religious prohibition, still less revulsion (the influential Alexandrine School was reputed to have practised live dissection), as a simple lack of interest in what the body might evidence. Where previously physicians had relied on the magisterial interpretation of canonical texts, most notably those of Galen, or on observation of the body's surfaces, the empiricists of the Enlightenment believed that in the investigation of the interior of the corpse they revealed the secrets of life. Medical illustrations of the period are full of images of the removal of the mystifying veil of the flesh and the opening up of enclosed spaces. In a reappraisal of man's relationship with death what was revealed was both the truth of life and a new understanding of disease. 'It is in death that disease and life speak their truth' (Foucault 1973: 143). Death was no longer seen as an external threat but as an inherent property of the pathological body (ibid.: 142). The way to study disease, then, was through the dead body.

Death itself had become the key to knowledge. But where contemporary practitioners of the discipline of anatomy believed themselves to be engaged in an uncovering of existent 'truths', almost in the sense of *alethia* (the re-membering of the real), Foucault understands their endeavours to be the active construction of knowledge. It is the anatomo-clinical gaze, concentrated on the corpse, that constructs the category of the morbid, and indeed of the normal. Just, then, at the point at which the epistemological division between life and death is problematised, the dualism of the normal and the pathological gains currency. At the same time, the management of pathological states which grew out of the investigation of the dead served to map and delimit the boundaries of the individual body. Modern medicine, as opposed to the abstract classificatory systems it finally replaced in the eighteenth century, was pre-eminently the science of the individual, a science which both constructs and privileges the normal body as an analytic framework and as an object of social enquiry. As Foucault claims, 'it is in [the] perception of death that the individual finds himself' (ibid.: 171). And what Foucault returns to again and again throughout his career is the way in which the discursive construction of the individual body, as an effect of the endless circulation of power and knowledge, provides the focus for the disciplinary and regulatory techniques practised upon the individual as person. That is not to say that such techniques are to be cast in a negative light, and in that respect there is nothing to distinguish between the discourse of health care as beneficence and, for example, the discourse of law as punitive. Both are regulatory practices.

Now although the brief outline which I have given of the medical model and of aspects of Foucault's explanation in *The Birth of the Clinic* for the rise of modern medicine both privilege the empirical gaze, the bodies of which they speak are not of the same order. Where for the former, the biological body and soul are constructed as radically disjunct, for Foucault the body is a site of intersection, not so much between the mundane and transcendental, as between power, the corporeal flesh and the individual as subject to and of truth(s). I will return to that later, but will mark here that neither formula signals any awareness that male and female bodies may be constructed not simply as different, but are differentially constructed. This is all the more surprising in Foucault's case where the consistent reference to the power/knowledge regime makes it difficult to understand how he could overlook the persistence of male dominance as a social form throughout the space and time of his enquiry. Nonetheless, a feminist analysis shares with Foucault a critique of biological determinism, which posits a given fixed body of health, and of the human sciences such as medicine and psychology in so far as they act as forms of social control. Moreover, both feminists and Foucauldians see the body, and more specifically sexuality, as central to the interplay of power and resistance. Once it is acknowledged that truth itself is constructed not discovered, then specific interests – be they racial, class, sexual or gender – pertaining to the dominant agents of discursive power must clearly affect the content of that truth. In illustration, I propose to look again at the way in which differential constructions of the body are by no means innocent of gender interests.

In order to have a better understanding of the discourse around the female body, I shall turn to its most prominent focus, not simply in the area of health care but in more general cultural representation, where women have been either invisible as a separate category or traditionally positioned as reproducers, regardless of any individual intention or ability to exercise that capacity. At the most reductive level, women have been seen as little more than baby machines; and even when the derogatory valuation of that is put aside, it does seem to express a self-evident truth that the reproductive role is more properly that of the woman than the man. The simple expediency of providing sperm has been represented as hardly bearing comparison with the long process of conception and gestation which is actually internal to women's bodies. That the reproductive body stands for something essentially female, and that to be valorised as a life-giver just is to be valorised as a woman, has been taken as a biological given. Nonetheless, that body has no stable history, and the valuation put on it has been consistent only in so far as it has been consistently less than that given to the male body. Moreover, whichever conception of the self is privileged – as either a transcendental attribute of mind or as fully embodied – the selfhood of women, whether it is characterised as deficient or excessive, is always inferior, incapable of full independent agency.

In the late twentieth century, medical literature around reproduction, intended for popular consumption, often goes to great lengths to stress that the process and associated responsibilities

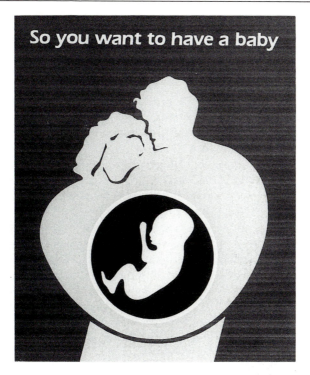

So you want to have a baby

Figure 1.2   Front cover of *So You Want to Have a Baby* (Serono booklet 1992). Courtesy Serono Ltd.

are not those of women alone. Where the emphasis is on pregnant couples rather than on pregnant women (Kirejczyk and van der Ploeg 1992), the archetypal image is that peddled by a commercial booklet *So You Want to Have a Baby* (Neuberg 1992), which has been widely available in family planning and fertility clinics in Great Britain. The front cover illustration depicts a heterosexual couple, the smaller woman merging into the man's arms, and the exposed foetus *in utero* overlapping both bodies (Figure 1.2). The text inside, which outlines the normal process of fertility and explains the various types of investigation and treatments for infertility, is clearly addressed to the woman partner alone, but stresses nevertheless: 'Your husband should always be encouraged to attend the clinic with you as *you are a unit* and the "problem" [infertility] is a joint one' (ibid.: 7, my emphasis). Despite citing a 40 per-cent incidence of male factor infertility (ibid.: 30),

however, the onus of undergoing exploratory and invasive exam-
inations falls squarely on the woman. Whereas she is expected to
undergo a full gynaecological examination on her first clinic visit,
the equivalent processing of the man 'can usually be deferred until
it becomes obvious that there is a significant male infertility factor'
(ibid.: 10). Similarly, even when oligospermia or azoospermia has
been identified as the proximate cause of infertility, the 'treatments' available – aside from such minor modifications of male
behaviour as the avoidance of constrictive underwear, hot baths,
excessive alcohol intake or overweight – are located in the body
of the fertile partner, the woman. Where artificial insemination
by husband is inappropriate, the treatment of choice[8] is increasingly likely to be not the equally technically simple procedure of
donor insemination, but the complex, invasive and often ineffective procedure of in vitro fertilisation (IVF), which involves both
chemical and mechanical intervention into the woman's body.
Finally, although blame for infertility should be imputed to neither
sex, it is revealing to compare the booklet's attitude to potentially
adverse factors. While men are merely advised to 'remove known
environmental causes' (my emphasis) such as those listed above
(ibid.: 32), the author becomes mildly chastising when age is a
secondary consideration: 'more and more women are sadly
delaying their attempt to start a family until well into their 30s
and even early 40s because they feel committed to their careers'
(ibid.: 3).

The overall impression then is both that women are and should
be more implicated in the reproductive process, and that they are
somehow likely to fall short in face of those responsibilities. What
is interesting is that, although the recognition of men's biological
involvement may be stressed and their social involvement
normalised, it is women's bodies which are manipulable. The
underlying subtext of such representations is that women themselves are incomplete without men, and that even their identities
as mothers cannot stand alone. Their bodies are, after all, just
bodies, involved necessarily in the processes of procreation, but
not quite capable of sustaining full personhood. That women
should entertain independent goals and desires is scarcely
addressed.

Even more alarming, as I shall go on to show, is that what the
new reproductive technologies of the late twentieth century have
done increasingly, though by no means uniquely, is to fragment

the female body itself. The wholeness of one's being-in-the-world is undermined in two directions. First, the reproductive organs of women are referred to as discrete entities to be directly managed. The woman as a person plays little or no part, but is obscured as an intentional agent by the clinical concentration on a set of functional norms. Kathryn Pauly Morgan, for example, sees this as an example of sexual objectification in which: '[a]n individual woman experiences the fragmentation of the integrated experience of fertility as she, personally, comes to be seen as a "difficult" assemblage of organs and processes, some of which may be malfunctioning' (1989: 74). Second, the status of the foetus or embryo, even the pre-conceptus at times, is characterised as free-floating, independent, radically other than the mother herself. This is evident both in medical and legal discourse where the foetus is treated as a subject in its own right (Martin 1991; Sherwin 1992: 105–7), and more dramatically in visual imagery (Petchesky 1987). At best, the mother's body – and this is an idea which has been recirculated throughout medical history – is just a container, a bounded space within which certain processes occur. At worst, the maternal body may be effaced altogether. The complete move is well illustrated by E. Ann Kaplan in her analysis of the mother in popular culture. Citing the impact made by Lennart Nilsson's 1965 photographic collection *A Child is Born*, she comments:

> The foetus is presented as already a full-blown subject, a baby, rather than an entity *in process*. The emphasis is all on the baby-to-be read back into the zygote. Further, the fact that this is all taking place in the mother's body is … ignored. The photos have no boundary to them that might represent the limit of the mother's womb or fallopian tubes. The mother is simply not a part of anything.
>
> (Kaplan 1992: 204)

What these discourses show, as I shall discuss in more detail in Chapter 6, is the way in which feminine ontology is intrinsically compromised. Given that women are stereotypically constructed in terms of their biological and more particularly reproductive bodies, at the same time those bodies express little real sense of personal presence. Corporeality and absence are coincidental.

As I have already outlined, that paradox is scarcely peculiar to the twentieth century, and may be traced back at least as far as the European Enlightenment when the Cartesian *cogito* 'I think therefore I am' signalled the privileging of mind over body. The self-present, self-authorising subject became *he* who could successfully transcend his own body to take up a position of pure reason uncontaminated by the untrustworthy experience of the senses. And once the supposedly objective, rational 'view from nowhere' became the new standard for human endeavour, women's pre-existing social disadvantages were philosophically reinforced. Although both sexes clearly do have material bodies, only women, because of their more intimate association with reproduction, were seen as intrinsically unable to transcend them. In the dominant discourse – and there are of course always competing counter-currents – that mind/body dichotomy is itself closely interwoven with a similar split between culture and nature (de Beauvoir 1968; Hekman 1990). Women were, in other words, more strongly linked to the natural processes of nurturance, and by extension to Mother Nature herself. It should not be supposed that the juxtaposition between male and female principles, nor even the positive valuation given to the male side, is unique to modernity. The ancient Greeks, for instance, operated similar systems, but what was new in post-Enlightenment (scientific) thought was the increasingly hierarchical structure of the by now familiar opposition between male–culture and female–nature. The more positively valued aspects of nurturance were overridden by the rationalist characterisation of nature as wild and chaotic, but nevertheless fundamentally machine-like and potentially controllable (Hekman 1990: 114). In directing its attention to the mastery of the natural world, and given the close identification of the female with nature, the scientific project of the Enlightenment may be conceptualised as inherently hostile to women.[9] Moreover the discursive circulation of both those heavily gendered binaries has grounded a belief in the deficient moral capabilities of the female sex.

In being somehow more fully embodied than men, women have been characterised simply as less able to rise above uncontrollable natural processes and passions and therefore disqualified from mature personhood. It is as though bodies could somehow interfere with moral thought, instructing the mind, rather than the other way round as is the case with men. Losing control of oneself is to a large degree synonymous with losing control of, or having no control over, one's body. In scientific and medical discourse in particular, it is quintessentially a feminine rather than masculine trait, predictable and tolerated in women, but sufficient to disqualify us from the mental self-governance necessary to (rational) moral agency. Normative constructions of medical syndromes such as hysteria and its modern-day counterparts, anorexia nervosa and bulimia, are strongly gender-linked, and suggest someone who is in need of control by others.[10] In contrast, any man who does experience or manifest the characteristic symptoms of such syndromes, far from being confirmed in his gender identity, is likely to be deemed deficient in his masculinity.

For women losing control is only to be expected. Though past explanations, such as the concept of the wandering womb, have been superseded by new constructions of female disorder, sophisticated medical references to hormones, pre-menstrual tension, menopausal irritability and the like are no less rooted in an essentialist view of women's bodies and women's nature.[11] And what these specifically female maladies – unmatched by male equivalents – serve to justify is paternalistic intervention on the grounds of both medical and moral incompetency. In consequence, the health-care encounter is a paradigmatic site of male power concerned with the control of a largely feminine irrationality which results not just from the compromised rationality caused by the pain and anxiety of ill health, but is supposedly rooted in our very natures. In turn, that nature relies upon particular biological constructions of the female body. More particularly it is the area of reproduction which grounds the differential account of male and female agency.

Not surprisingly the post-Enlightenment emphasis on difference, focused on the binary of male mind and female body, extended to the biological differences between bodies themselves. It is strange then to find, as Thomas Laqueur has argued, that the widespread adoption and acknowledgement of a two-sex model, male and female, for the body was a fairly late feature of medical and more specifically anatomical knowledge. According to Laqueur, what was in play prior to 1800 was what he refers to as the one-sex model in which the bodies of women were understood, not just on an abstract level, but in material terms too, to be simply inferior versions of the male body (Laqueur 1990a: 25–6). Following the model of the reproductive organs proposed by Galen (*De semine* II, 5; 1992: 189–91), early anatomists such as Berengario, in his *Isagogae breves* (1522; 1959, trans. Lind), ignored the detail of clinical observation and provided highly schematic illustrations which uncritically testified to the 'truth' of classical medical knowledge. In contrast, in the major work by Vesalius, for example, *De humani corporis fabrica* (1543; Saunders *et al.* 1950), which set the standard for empirical anatomy for decades to come, the images are supposedly drawn from life. Nonetheless, despite their representational sophistication they perpetuate an entrenched orthodoxy in which the female generative organs are isomorphic with those of the male.

That the 'truth' of anatomy had moved from text-based authority to that of the clinical gaze made little difference: what Vesalius and his followers continued to see was a one-sex body in which the configuration of organs might be different, but in which structure and form, and indeed the names given to the apparently corresponding male and female parts, was the same. The internal location of the female testes, as the ovaries were called, or of the penile vagina (Figure 1.3) was explained as a lower stage of anatomical development and was consistent with the contemporary discourse of female inferiority. Though no one discourse enjoyed a monopoly, I would suggest that what the dominant images of female genitalia as the mirror of the male exposed was that medical knowledge was constructed to correspond to a philosophical truth. Women were not seen to be radically different and incommensurate with men, but simply imperfectly formed versions – both physically and ontologically – of the accepted standard, which was intrinsically male. They were, in other words, incorporated within the same, judged against a male ideal which they inevitably failed to express, and thereby devalued in their own right.[12]

And yet how could the gaze of Renaissance scientism represent the female body as a version of the male? We may allow for widespread resemblances in very general anatomy, but from the late modern viewpoint what appears as a gross anatomical distortion is that the reproductive organs in particular should be forced into a univisual perspective. Given that the practice of postmortem, as far as it had existed at all, was largely abandoned after the second century AD in favour of abstract speculation on the body, and that the teaching of anatomy became a reiteration of classical texts, it is understandable that for centuries the guesses, generalisations and plain prejudices of the early medical establishment should simply be reproduced unchanged. But more than that, with the advent of a new empirical approach it must appear that to a certain extent the tradition was not just unquestioned

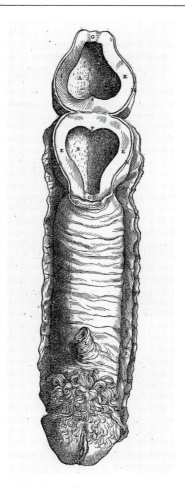

Figure 1.3 Andreas Vesalius: *De humani corporis fabrica. Lib. V,
fig. 27* (1543). 'Penile' uterus and vagina. Courtesy Wellcome
Institute Library, London

but unquestionable. In any case, although human dissection was
rarely practised in the intervening centuries, animals were occasionally still used without that making any apparent impact on
the strange and to our eyes incorrect mirroring by which the
female genitalia were explained. If, as Laqueur (1990a: 70)
outlines, there was, in effect, an enormous resistance to revising
the traditional models even after human anatomy was more

thoroughly explored in practice, then we must conclude that the need to uncover a particular truth about women outweighed any contrary empirical evidence.

Yet again, I want to be clear that I am not positing any pre-given morphology which it is simply the task of science to discover. It is not that a late modern version of truth should be preferred as more closely corresponding to reality, nor that it is any less mediated by contemporary discursive practices than that which it replaces. On the contrary, my position is postmodern in that it problematises truth/knowledge as a shifting and multiple construction determined only in as far as it expresses a more or less temporary alliance of intersecting forces. The experience of any 'underlying' reality is put aside, not because it does not exist, but because it is inaccessible in any prediscursive state. In any case, the interpretations which are being contested here are local and specific, and do not necessarily preclude the possibility of objectively real bodies. Moreover, though the body may always be seen as a text, it must be addressed in its concrete specificity, not as some immaterial abstraction. The point of my enquiry, then, is not to disparage some and privilege other readings of the body, but to question the cultural significance of how each came to be taken as true. The issue, as Foucault says, 'is not that everything is bad, but that everything is dangerous' (1982: 232). And that insight, as I shall show shortly in specific detail, inevitably involves a challenge to the practices of the body. For the moment, however, I shall continue to trace its differential construction. In contradistinction to any account of progress, what is of concern are precisely the ruptures and shifts that constitute a genealogy of the body.

Once again it should be remembered that there are always multiple and competing discourses that thwart any move to pin down a unified account of how the body has been historically constructed. Nonetheless, my intention for the moment is to trace the dominant and authorised forms, to look at the body as the focus of convention. Following, then, the historical model proposed by Laqueur, it is surely significant that the point at which evidence of bodily difference became undeniable, and indeed accepted as the new orthodoxy, was the point at which the mind/body split of the Enlightenment decisively shifted the parameters of subjectivity, and constructed personhood as other than the body. The universal isomorphic truth of the human body, expressed both in terms of sexual indifferentiation and of ontological unity, was displaced by the oppositional split of mind/body, male/female. At the same time, the natural world, which had traditionally been feminised, was made subject to control by science. The imagery of Nature unveiled before Science, of the body stripped of its fleshy protection and penetrated by the empirical gaze is strongly gender-linked (Jordanova 1980, 1989).

Once the body itself had been devalued by its disengagement from the controlling mind, then the explanation of female inferiority found new grounds, and one must suppose that the ideological interest in maintaining the premise that female bodies were imperfectly formed male ones was greatly weakened. Indeed, the concept of male-determined correspondences or sameness gave way to recognition of what was *other* than, and incommensurate with, the male. What is striking here, however, is the way in which the construction of the medical knowledge about gendered bodies moves between the standards of sameness and difference without in any sense revising the attribution of inferiority to the female form. Where once the female was simply represented as a deficient version of the male ideal, the new knowledge constructed women as radically different from men, but no less made relative to and devalued against a male standard. In other words, difference was recognised but the hierarchy was maintained.

Now all of this changing anatomical knowledge finds an echo in the differential way in which the very process of reproduction, as well as the genital organs themselves, have experienced a radical shift in perception. Just as the one-sex model of the body was dominant until the late eighteenth century, so women's specific part in reproduction was obscured by the insistence on the male as the progenitor of life. If women were morphologically inferior, then clearly their role in conception and even gestation could not be given serious credit. That is not to say that the classical authorities were in agreement as to how reproduction worked, but as both Maclean (1980) and Tuana (1988; 1993, chapter 7) amply illustrate, the common thread which links Aristotle to Galen was the determined downgrading of female agency in the reproductive processes. Where Galen allowed that conception involved the fusion of both male and female seed, of which the latter was simply less important, being colder and less active (*De semine* II, 2; 1992: 165–7), Aristotle's theory of one-seed gestation signalled a process wherein women played no real part, providing only the raw material to which the male sperma alone brought form (*De generatione animalium* 729a; 1953: 109). The material body was in effect the nutritional container for new life, but had little contribution to make to the principle of generation itself. This almost complete erasure of active female participation mirrors Aristotle's view that the active spirit was an exclusively male attribute, and it finds its analogue in Judaeo-Christian views of the creation. Almost two millennia later, a similar move reappeared in the doctrine of spermatic preformation which became the dominant model of procreation from around 1680 until near the end of the eighteenth century.

It was the belief of the Preformationists that all living things were created at the beginning, later generations being as it were enclosed within earlier ones. Given the lack of scientific instrumentation at the end of the seventeenth century either to confirm or nullify the material claims of the doctrine, the medical scientist Nicolaus Hartsoeker proposed and speculatively illustrated the existence within the sperm of a perfectly formed animalcule (Figure 1.4). In Hartsoeker's version, each sperm contained in effect a minute but completed homunculus which was simply activated by being implanted in the female womb. In other words, there was no new generation in nature but only an increase in size and hardness of parts that were already present (Tuana 1988: 51–5; 1993: 148). Although a similar theory of ovist preformation slightly predated and was for a time co-terminous with the spermatic model, Tuana claims (1988: 53; 1993: 150) that it quickly fell from favour in the face of a competitor that favoured male primacy. What she does not consider is that although the ovists might seem to privilege maternal involvement, in fact in preferring, if not male, then divine provenance, they enacted the same denial of maternal origin and substance as their rivals. The theory of preformation as such did not long survive past the end of the eighteenth century, but it is worth noting that even now a similar image of increase appears in at least one major anatomy text. The Embryology section of *Gray's Anatomy*, originally published in 1858 and consistently updated since, continues to illustrate the development of the foetus from the fourth to the tenth lunar month as though it entailed nothing more than a lengthening or increase in parts (Williams 1995: 332). In a similar way, the imagery employed by anti-abortionists regularly suggests the

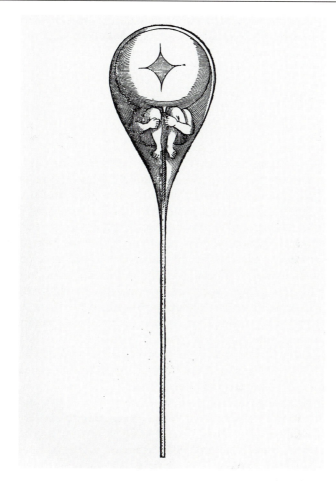

Figure 1.4   Nicolaus Hartsoeker: *Essai de diotropique* (1694).
Human spermatozoon containing animalcule. Courtesy Wellcome
Institute Library, London

presence at all stages post-conception, of a fully formed infant
body (Petchesky 1987).

However women's bodies have been downgraded, one recur-
ring explanation of their inferiority, supported by classical and
pre-modern humoral theory, is that, unlike men, they lacked heat
and were instead excessively cold and moist. The axiom that the
hottest things are the most perfect is unexplained in classical texts,

and nor is it clear just what it is that constitutes precisely women's coldness. Galen simply reiterates the truism behind such thinking when he writes:

> Now just as mankind is the most perfect of all the animals, so within mankind the man is more perfect than the woman, and the reason for his perfection is his excess of heat, for heat is Nature's primary instrument.
>
> (*De usu partium* 14, II, 299; 1968: 630)

In contrast to the male standard, female heat deficiency has been cited variously as the proximate reason why women were unable to produce fertile seed of their own, why their genitalia remained underdeveloped and internal, and why their brains simply did not function at the same level as those of males. Even when the one-sex model of gendered degrees of perfection was being abandoned, however, the notion of women's lesser temperature remained; though according to Maclean a functional explanation had become commonly accepted by the end of the sixteenth century: '[woman's] colder metabolism causes her to consume ("burn up") food less fast, thus leaving residues of fat and blood which are necessary for the nutriment of the foetus and for the eventual production of milk' (1980: 34). Nonetheless, when unused this otherwise productive residue offered a continuing explanation of female psychological inferiorities.

In monthly menstruation both the loss of vital blood and the confirmation of an internal build-up of noxious waste material further underlined the dissipation of women's bodily vigour and their reduced intellectual capacity. Moreover, the very sign of fertility, the menses, has been regarded as evidence of women's inherent lack of control of the body and, by extension, of the self. In other words, women, unlike the self-contained and self-containing men, leaked; or, as Grosz claims: 'women's corporeality is inscribed as a mode of seepage' (1994: 203). The issue throughout Western cultural history has been one of female lack of closure,[13] a negative coding all too evident in one of Sartre's many derogations of the gross materiality of the female body: '[t]he obscenity of the feminine sex is that of everything which "gapes open"' (1958: 613). The indeterminacy of body boundaries challenges that most fundamental dichotomy between self and other, unsettling ontological certainty and threatening to undermine the basis on which the knowing self establishes control.

I shall mark here only the paradox that while women are represented as more wholly embodied than men, that embodiment is never complete nor secure. And nowhere perhaps is female excess more evident and more provocative of male anxiety than in reproduction. The capacity to be simultaneously both self and other in pregnancy, which is the potential of every woman, is the paradigm case of breached boundaries.

In a nexus of related ideas, the concept of female pollution is strong. Where Aristotle simply asserted the heat/cold dichotomy as the basis of women's generative and intellectual inferiority (*De generatione animalium* 766a; 1953: 391), Galen attempted to provide a physiological explanation according to which male and female embryos were formed in crucially different ways. While the male embryo resulted from a fusion of seeds involving one from the right-hand ovary of the mother, the female embryo relied on a seed from the left-hand ovary (Figure 1.5). The importance of this distinction, as Galenic anatomy showed, was that though the blood supply to the right ovary passed first through a kidney where it was cleansed, that to the left ovary had not yet done so and was, as Galen puts it, 'uncleansed, full of residues, watery and serous' (*De usu partium* 14, II, 306; 1968: 635). As a result, female embryos were already marked *in utero* by waste material and impure blood, and were therefore subsequently unable to generate heat. And the discursive construction of this quasi-scientific explanation so perfectly served to support cultural expectations of women's inferiority that it went unchallenged well into the Renaissance – even after the wider practice of human dissection might have been expected to reveal that Galen's claims were based on what a later age saw as anatomical inaccuracies.

Again the final abandonment of the old orthodoxy could be linked to the post-Enlightenment devaluation of bodies in general. Once mind became the superior power, and the real mark of human self-consciousness, male dominance shifted its justificatory claims. Far from occupying a secondary position in relation to reproduction, women's bodies and consequently women's identities were now reconstructed as essentially different from those of men, and moreover, focused on the maternal function. This is not to say of course that men ceded material power over reproduction but that their own subjectivities were expressed elsewhere. Flesh-and-blood bodies, and their particular capacities and problems, were the mark of the feminine.

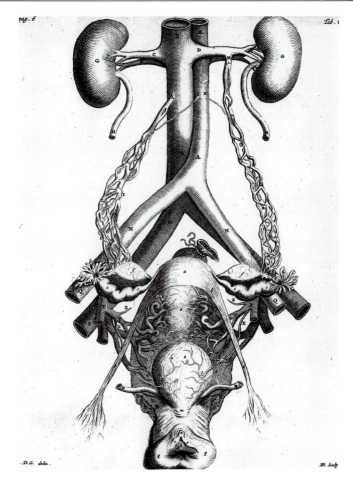

Figure 1.5 Regnerus de Graaf: *De mulierum organis generationi inservientibus tractatus novus* (1672). Female reproductive organs showing differential supply of blood to left and right ovaries. Courtesy Wellcome Institute Library, London

And yet once more there is a curious contradiction: on the one hand feminine immanence, the being-in-the-body that precluded mental maturity, and on the other a certain ongoing insubstantiality about the very things, largely in the field of reproduction, which are cited as the grounds for women's inability to transcend their bodies. This has become increasingly evident in the context

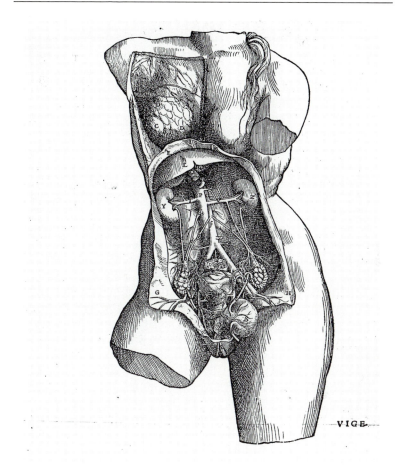

Figure 1.6 Andreas Vesalius: *De humani corporis fabrica* (1543).
Upper female torso. Courtesy Wellcome Institute Library, London

of New Reproductive Technologies, those strange postmodern
effects of dispersal on embodied selves; but, interestingly, insubstantiality seems to have been a factor all along. In illustration I
want to look again at the renaissance of anatomy in the fifteenth
to seventeenth centuries, at the time when, as Laqueur claims,
the one-sex model was still predominant. What contemporary
representations show is that where male bodies are all structure
and solidity, women's bodies are dematerialised, and more often

represented in terms of surfaces and internal spaces. The corresponding plates of dissected male and female torsos from Vesalius' *Fabrica* – extensively copied by de Valverde and Vidius, for example – are composed to show on the one hand the dense unified structure of male musculature and skeletal form, but on the other the smooth surface skin and relative interior emptiness of the female body in which the organs of reproduction appear unsupported (Figure 1.6). While the one suggests the very presence of masculine being in the world, the other is insubstantial. The female body reveals its inner secrets to the anatomical gaze as something quite apart from surface impressions. It is as though the inner and outer body are somehow divided against each other, and there is no 'whole' woman to know.

Just as the inner and outer body of the female are represented as discontinuous, so too it is comparatively rare in medical illustration of any period to find images which show the embryo/foetus as having any essential connection with the maternal body. The foetus is portrayed either as decontextualised, within the uterus but without the body – and this is increasingly common in historically recent representations – or it is located within the maternal environment, but as seemingly separate and autonomous, finding temporary shelter and nurturance rather than connectedness. In pre-modern representations, the foetus *in utero* was invariably drawn schematically as a fully formed infant standing or crouching in its own space, awaiting as it were release into an outer world (Figure 1.7). Although later illustrations provided a somewhat more realistic image of the foetus, the suggestion of self-sufficiency remained. In a plate from the eighteenth century, for example, depicting the opened-up pregnant body of a woman, the sense of disconnection is powerful, for not only is the infant body highly developed and seemingly independent in that it can be removed from the womb, but the mother herself shows no concern at her interior burden. To all intents her body is simply a container, contingently filled, but essentially empty, and the woman as person is marked by absence (Figure 1.8).

Such images are by no means unusual in their implicit fragmentation of the embodied experience of pregnancy, a move that is further developed in representations where the female body is absent in its entirety. In these the foetus may float in a disembodied uterus, anchored by the umbilical cord, but having connection only to an abstract source of life. In many seventeenth-

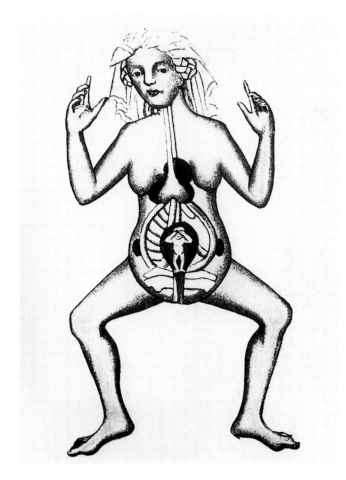

Figure 1.7 Gravida in manuscript miniature from *Leinzig Codex 1122* (*c.* 1400). Courtesy Wellcome Institute Library, London

and eighteenth-century texts intended for the teaching of midwifery, for example, a hand pushed up through the vagina, and emblematic of the external world, provides the only signifier of connection (Figure 1.9). A similar form of imaging has found its apotheosis in later twentieth-century reproductive technologies where both verbal and visual representation reinforce the dis-integration of women's bodies. It is not simply a radical disjunct between outer and inner, but the effective disappearance of the

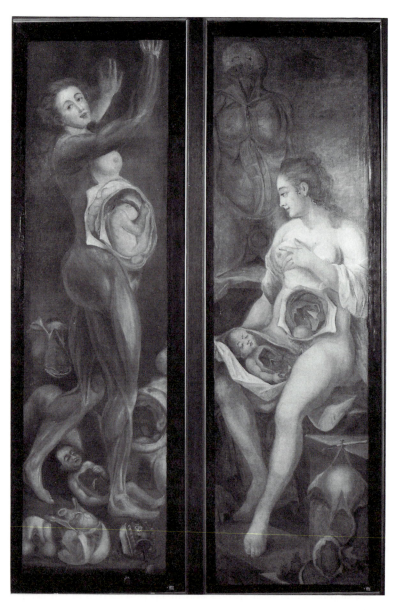

Figure 1.8. J.F. Gautier d'Agoty (eighteenth century). Anatomical painting of female figures with infants and a foetus *in utero*. Courtesy Wellcome Institute Library, London

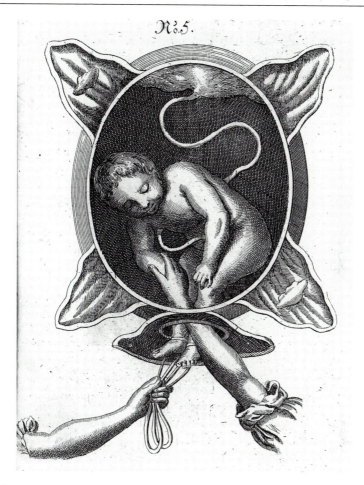

Figure 1.9.   Justine Siegmund: *Die konigl. preussische und chur-brandenb* (1723). Foetus being removed from womb; illustration in a midwifery manual. Courtesy Wellcome Institute Library, London

whole body/whole person as such. There is little sense in current medical literature of the woman as intentional agent, but only of disembodied and discrete reproductive processes. What is represented is not the mother, but at best fragmentary bits of her. Even in very early stages of pregnancy, the shadowy images of ultrasound serve to construct the foetus as an entity in its own right. The rest is space and silence.

The essential lack of substance, the quasi-emptiness of the female body is a culturally recurrent theme which seems to have survived other shifts in the perception of female anatomy. It pervades, for example, at least one strand of classical medical discourse which remained influential over many centuries. As early as Plato the womb was likened to an animal capable of independent movement within the body cavity (*Timaeus* 91a; 1965: 120), and by the first century AD uterine displacement (the 'wandering womb'), cited as the cause of a range of symptoms, was a well-established phenomenon. A common precipitating factor was held to be lack of sexual intercourse, so that Aretaeus of Cappadocia was able to claim that widows, elderly virgins and adolescents were especially prone to the disorder. The characterisation of the perceived syndrome in medieval texts as '*suffocatio matricis*' expressed the idea that the sensory disturbances, or so-called hysteria, were the result of a form of internal suffocation. The cause was held to be either organic, with the womb itself rising upwards to compress breathing, or alternatively it was due to the pressures of unexpelled menstrual fluid flooding the brain (Jacquart and Thomasset 1988). Two major markers of female bodies, internal emptiness and leakiness, come together here in the explanatory accounts. And not surprisingly, the accepted cure for this supposedly intrinsic female aberrance was entry into a sexual relationship with a man.

The paradox of immanence and lack of substance is paralleled by another contradiction in that, although it was the internal *retention* of the organs of generation which marked the female in the one-sex model, there was no corresponding sense in which the male body was therefore emptier. On the contrary, as one seventeenth-century text, cited by Laqueur (1990a: 141), argues, transsexualism from men to women was impossible as there was insufficient room inside the male body into which a penis could invert.[14] Again it might be expected that once the one-sex model, in which the female body is an inferior and underdeveloped version of the male, had been transformed by a new focus on sexual differentiation, that the recognition of distinct female reproductive morphology would give new substantiality to women's bodies. Certainly the uterus, vagina and above all the ovaries took on enormous consequence as the determinants of female behaviour, and indeed were the site of brutal medical intervention in the interests of promoting acceptable femininity, but the focus remained nevertheless dis-integrated and essentially reductionist.

The metonymic circulation of specific body parts simply emphasises the absence of the body itself. And in the discourse of psychoanalysis too, which Foucault (1979) characterised as the paradigmatic human science, the visual, and by now material, absence of the penis has been taken as the defining factor of femininity. Women are castrated men, their bodies marked by lack, and what is hidden is just a hole. Where for men, the penis/phallus, real and symbolic, has become the very signifier of presence and of wholeness, women, having no thing, are in consequence nothing. In a scathing critique of Freud's analysis of women, Luce Irigaray attributes to him the view that '*Nothing to be seen is equivalent to having no thing. No being and no truth*' (1985a: 48). As Irigaray makes clear, it is not just that the body is constructed as absence, but that women themselves are ontologically out of order. The leaks and flows in the corpus are – as I shall explore in more detail later – the markers of a far more troubling lack of form: a resistance to closure which threatens disruption ultimately to the whole structuration of the Western logos.

Initially, then, these brief snapshots of women's bodies, contradictory and often discontinuous as they are, should serve to alert us to the dangers of regarding biology as given. Though we are familiar with the view that holds health to be both a normative and normalising term, any worthwhile analysis needs to go further to problematise the corporeal body itself. As women, our being-in-the-world cannot be understood by reference to any fixed or essential bodily core. Ways of seeing and ways of knowing are not predicated on a reality somehow beyond discourse, but are deeply implicated in the construction of bodies and selves. It is interesting in this light to consider Maclean's explanation of how Renaissance commentaries, faced with both a continuing respect for Classical medical authority and new empirical technology, struggled 'to maintain a synthetic outlook with the help of ingenious and sometimes makeshift strategies of interpretation' (Maclean 1980: 44). But there is surely more to it than that. As Foucault (1980) has demonstrated, power and knowledge are productive and indissolubly linked forces; and though Foucault himself fails to remark it, in patriarchal society the dominant discourses are those which consolidate and extend the male social order.[15] Accordingly, though there is *in reality* no fixed referent, the male body (in its own various constructions) is posited as the natural standard against which the female body is measured and valued – as inferior, as different, as insubstantial, as absent.

THE DISCIPLINARY BODY

Having once established the historically specific and differential construction of the body, it remains to enquire into what Foucault calls the practices of the body. If our perception relies on a variable discursive artefact, then how is that perception put into play and acknowledged as the truth of our being? Alongside the various empirical discourses of the body – anatomy, physiology and genetics, for example – which constitute the life sciences, late modernity has seen the emergence of a proliferation of human sciences like sociology, anthropology and psychoanalysis. Now it may appear that where the former set are concerned with explanation and functional analysis, and the latter with normative standards of human being and behaviour, they constitute what Rosi Braidotti, taking a Foucauldian reading, calls 'a division of labour' in the discourses of the body. She goes on:

> on the one hand the body is simply another object of knowledge, an empirical object among others: an organ-ism, the sum of its organic parts, an assembly of detachable organs. . . . On the other hand, no body can be reduced to the sum of its organic components: the body still remains the site of the transcendence of the subject, and as such it is the condition of possibility for all knowledge. Foucault concludes that the body is an empirical-transcendental double.
>
> (Braidotti 1991b: 358)

Now, although I would agree that Foucault writes the body in both its materiality and its ontology, it is not entirely clear from Braidotti's exposition that he is concerned to unsettle the implicit dualism which she notes. As I have already remarked, the corporeal body is for Foucault inseparable from the power practised upon it and from the selfhood which grounds the knowing and known subject. In consequence, subjectivity cannot be said to be transcendent but is marked by the continual process of the body. Indeed, Braidotti herself is elsewhere consistently and explicitly concerned with the embodiment of the modern subject. Moreover, the split between social and biosciences is not left unproblematised as she seems to indicate, but is implicitly deconstructed by Foucault's painstaking analysis, in *The Birth of the Clinic*, of the anatomo-clinical body as the site of emergent individuality, and again in the introductory volume of *The History of Sexuality* where the construction of the sexual body stands as the truth of the embodied subject. In contradistinction to Braidotti's remark that the human sciences are 'connected to the question of an ethics or a politics; which is not necessarily the case for the "hard", or for the biomedical sciences' (ibid.), the point emerging from Foucauldian analytics is that in the production of truths there is no distinction to be made between empirical and normative disciplines. Rather, the so-called hard sciences are intermeshed with disciplinary practices. And given the contention that there can be no pure empiricism, as a genealogy of the body must surely show, I would argue that it is in the episteme and practice of biomedicine that 'factual' knowledge is most clearly complicit with both material and discursive mechanisms of control.

In Foucault's terms, the embodied being of the individual is both subject and subjected in that the knowing self is simultaneously constructed by that which he knows. I shall not further develop here Foucault's analysis of subjectivity, which engages with both the external technologies of domination in earlier work, and increasingly with the technologies of the self in later work, but note that throughout it is in the context of the sexuate body that the subject is constituted. His concern therefore is to ask:

> how it is in a society like ours, sexuality is not simply a means of reproducing the species, the family, and the individual? Not simply a means to obtain pleasure and enjoyment? How has sexuality come to be considered the privileged place where our deepest 'truth' is read and expressed? For that is the essential fact: Since Christianity, the Western world has never ceased saying: 'To know who you are, know what your sexuality is.'
>
> (1988: 110–11)

Indeed, so central is this consideration to his work that he sees the manifest and experienced human body as though saturated with sex. Accordingly, when he comes to analyse those powers which construct the person, it is most usually in terms of the forces which operate within sexuate meaning. How each person knows him or herself both as an individual and as a member of the social body is determined, then, less by the grand parameters of race, class, gender and so on, than by the specific and local way in which sexual identity is constructed and practised.

Perhaps one of Foucault's most notable insights has been to assert the productivity of modern power over against the repressive hypothesis which characterises power only as that which says 'no'. That is not to say that there are no negative effects, but rather that both models must circulate simultaneously. Far from imposing a single unitary discourse which works by exclusion and prohibition, the power/knowledge complex conceptualised by Foucault incites and mobilises a proliferation of effects. In *The History of Sexuality*, volume 1, for example, he shows how the 'perverse' sexualities of late modernity are constructed and exposed through a variety of techniques which continually multiply the discourses of the body while at the same time inserting them into patterns of normativity. In just such a way, what Foucault calls bio-power – that is, the power over life – operates by reaching into the private pleasures of individuals to liberate new public practices which constitute in effect systems of control. In other words, the local relations of sexuality emerge as the basis of new strategies which shape the social body by acting on the bodies of individuals. Power operates then in two highly interrelated spheres to produce and control both the docile body of the individual described in terms of its utility, efficiency and intelligibility, and the species body which grounds a bio-politics of population concerned with 'propagation, births and mortality, the level of health, life expectancy and longevity' (Foucault 1979: 139). The disciplines centred on the individual and the regulatory controls on population, which converge in directing the 'performances of the body, with attention to the processes of life' (ibid.: 139), constitute what Foucault calls a 'great technology of power' in which the deployment of sexuality is the most important element (ibid.: 140).

All this, as I have noted before, is elucidated without specific reference to gender, or to the differential power relationship between men and women, even though Foucault is well aware that the forces of bio-power operate largely over the female body. He lists (ibid.: 103–4) four specific focal points of power/knowledge, all of which manifest in familial contexts, and two of which also directly concern women: the 'hysterization of women's bodies' and the 'socialization of procreative behaviour'.[16] Nonetheless, the specificity of sexual difference remains untheorised, and Foucault fails to acknowledge that the techniques of domination which in the modern age serve capitalism are also implicated in the ongoing construction of patriarchy. There is no sense that gender has any especial significance in the deployment of power nor, as I have argued above, that the materiality of male and female bodies is of a different order. In Foucauldian terms, power operates as it were independently of its sexed agents, as an almost abstract force which differentially impacts on women in a non-necessary way. As a result many feminists have argued that Foucault is at best gender-indifferent and therefore of limited use to the feminist project, or at worst deliberately phallocentric in his concerns. As Linda Singer puts it: 'By failing to leave a place for a discourse of women's difference, the effect of Foucault's textual strategies is to reconstitute self-effacing masculinity as a unitary voice of authority' (1993: 157). Nonetheless, whilst I would agree that Foucault's analysis is flawed by his gender omissions, his deconstructive approach to the episteme of the body and to power is a stepping-stone of great significance to feminism in the contestation of the devaluation of women.

What I am suggesting is that Foucault's overall concern to write a non-essentialist and yet fully material account of the body is just that which grounds a particular form of feminist endeavour. We must envisage a two-fold analysis in which, alongside specific considerations of sexual difference, it makes sense to establish that all bodies are constructed by a combination of disciplinary and regulatory powers. In so far as both female and male bodies are inscribed by similar discursive and institutional modes of control, there is an area of overlap in which Foucault may legitimately centre his enquiry. Moreover, although the body to which he refers is largely unmarked by gender, it must not be forgotten that it is also crossed and mediated by other quasi-structural, but in reality equally discursive, categories, such as class, ethnicity, (dis)ability and sexual preference. All of these may both bind and separate women and men. With those provisos in mind, and the recognition that female bodies are never the exclusive target of regulatory forces, it is nonetheless also necessary 'to explore how meanings, particularly representations of gender, are mobilized within the operations of power to produce asymmetrical relations amongst subjects' (McNay 1992: 35). In other words, what is at issue for feminism is how any body becomes en-gendered as feminine or masculine. Indeed, given the non-accessibility of 'pure' corporeality, sex and gender can no longer be seen as epistemically discontinuous, and appeal to an authentic female body may be no less theoretically implausible than is gender essentialism. Despite that caution, however, to experience oneself and be experienced by others as a woman is to take up a particular bodily identity which grounds political action as a woman. Though far from essentialist, that identity is not yet reducible to the politically strategic, for if, as Foucault claims, power is ubiquitous, then in the performance of the body as sexed there may be no other choice. Nevertheless, what feminism can take from Foucault is the notion that the relations of power are 'matrices of transformation' (Foucault 1979: 99), which may always be susceptible to local resistance and to redistribution. The archaeological project of discovering alternative systems of thought profoundly disturbs and deflates the putative inevitability of patriarchal domination.

I have already looked at some discontinuities in the discursive construction of the female body, but what is the nature of the technologies of power which do not simply produce and maintain sexed behaviour, but are complicit in the very construction of the sexed body itself? Above all, power circulates in the procedures of normalisation by which, on the one hand, the body is inscribed with meaning (the intelligible body) and, on the other, rendered manageable (the useful/manipulable body) (Foucault 1977a: 136). Together these two modes constitute the docile body which 'may be subjected, used, transformed, and improved' (ibid.). The insertion of bodies into systems of utility, whether at the level of the individual or of the population – and each concerns here both capitalism and patriarchy – devolves on forms of power that are localised over the singular body, and that rely not on brute force but on quasi-voluntary acquiescence. The disciplinary and regulatory techniques practised on the body exemplify the productive nature of power in that they not only set up systems of control, but also call forth new desires and institute new normativities. In this, the sciences of man, of which Foucault characterises modern medicine as the first example and psychoanalysis as its preeminent form, are exemplary in that they constitute the individual in terms of a series of norms, while at the same time inviting the subject to produce truths about herself. It is not simply that 'the female body became a medical object *par excellence*' (Foucault 1988, 'Power and sex': 115), but that the gaze is complemented by a complex mesh of techniques of self-surveillance and confession. The clinical encounter is a paradigmatic site for the technologies of the body which both shape and control. Moreover, given that in Foucault's account certain practices may operate in a gender-specific manner, a feminist analysis of systems of health care may usefully appropriate and extend his insights.

In the modern welfare state, though the face-to-face encounter may concentrate the power of the medical gaze, the effects of health care as a disciplinary regime can extend into the most private and personal aspects of life. The demand to know intimate details about the individual is a common feature of state bureaucracy, but is nowhere more apparent than in the transaction between the welfare claimant and the multifarious overseeing benefit agencies. In recent years, the trend in Great Britain has been towards various forms of self-certification to replace in-person interview and examination; but far from liberating the claimant from an authoritarian and intrusive situation, the locus of power/knowledge has merely shifted to equally or additionally onerous forms of surveillance. The gaze now cast over the subject body is that of the subject herself. What is demanded of her is that she should police her own body, and report in intricate detail its failure to meet standards of normalcy; that she should render herself, in effect, transparent. At the same time the capillary processes of power reach ever deeper into the body, multiplying here not desire but the norms of function/dysfunction. As with confession, everything must be told, not by coercive extraction, but 'freely' offered up to scrutiny. The subject is made responsible, and thus all the more cautious and manageable, for her own success in obtaining state benefit. And should benefit be withheld then it may be attributed to a failure of reportage as much as to a denying external agency.

These particular modes of disciplinary practice are exemplified with great clarity in the procedures surrounding the benefit known as Disability Living Allowance (hereafter DLA). As a benefit directed towards a state of being that affects both men and women of all ages, classes, sexualities, ethnic groups and so on, DLA might seem to illustrate the general operation of power/knowledge in and over the body without specific relevance to gender. I have chosen it as an example, however, precisely because of the way in which disability imbricates conceptually with the wider issue of the existential disablement of the female body in Western society. Moreover the 'fact' of disablement is by no means gender-neutral, but, as state-sponsered research persistently shows, has a differential and greater impact on women.[17] Such surveys may be regarded as somewhat crude and much-contested indicators of the extent of disability, but nonetheless the demonstration of gender imbalance is widely accepted. As Martin *et al.* explain (1988: 24), the overall differential is produced because women on average live longer than men, and the prevalence of disability itself increases with age. On a purely empirical basis, then, there is good reason to view disability as overdetermined for women.

More important, however, in the context of my argument that female bodies are devalued in relation to the male and that they are the privileged target of disciplinary practices, is the way in which state-defined disability mirrors the phenomenological experience of women generally. Given that all women are positioned in relation to and measured against an inaccessible body ideal (in part determined by a universalised male body), the experience of female disablement as such may be seen as the further marginalisation of the already marginal. Where all women's experience of their corporeal integrity is generally under threat or inadequately addressed (Young 1990), then those who are additionally defined as disabled may find their bodily experience even more likely to be invalidated (Wendell 1992). In relation then to the 'whole' body of phenomenology women with disabilities are doubly dis-abled. It is worth noting too that in so far as disability/non-disability is positioned as a quasi-structural binary it impacts on the standards of normalcy operative for femininity itself. The insertion of female bodies into systems of normalisation, and the emergence of variable and hierarchical constructs of feminine identity, are highly mediated by such considerations.

None of this is intended to imply any pre-existing strategy to position 'empirical' disability as a peculiarly feminine condition, and indeed male claimants of DLA are subjected for the most part to the same extraordinary procedures as female ones. Nonetheless, in so far as the category of disability is constructed through such practices, it is so – as I have suggested elsewhere of the general signifier of ill health – as a condition that is engendered as feminine in terms of its implied dependency and passivity. Bearing in mind that the docile bodies produced by disciplinary techniques are an effect in every instance of power/knowledge, what is additionally striking about the shifting and heterogeneous set of conditions named as disability is that in its construction the disciplinary process is laid bare. And moreover, that heterogeneity is itself masked in the production of a regulatory category that operates as a homogeneous entity within the social body. Despite the emphasis given to what appear to be very singular determinations of a state of disability, it is in the very gestures of differentiation and individuation, as exemplified by the innumerable subdivisions of the questions posed on the DLA form, that the claimant is inserted into patterns of normalisation which grossly restrict individuality. Ultimately, what the technologies of the body effect, while appearing to incite the singular, is a set of co-ordinated and managed differences.

The specific benefit of DLA, which is intended for those who need help with 'personal care' or with 'getting around', was included in an extensive television and press campaign to promote a new user-friendly image for the Department of Social Security. Self-assessment plays a particularly large part in the claims procedure, although the limits of reliability of non-authoritative discourse are marked in that the subject's own report must be supplemented by statements from two other people who will be most usually health-care professionals. In other words, the gaze is multi-perspectival. What is remarkable about the claims pack (*DLA 580* 1993) sent to potential claimants is its sheer volume, in which four pages of initial notes are followed by twenty-eight pages of report, the vast majority of which consists of a detailed self-analysis of personal behaviour. The introductory instructions are quite clear about what is expected from claimant self-surveillance – '[t]he more you can tell us, the easier it is for us to get a clear picture of the type of help you need' (Section 2: 1) – and thus they suggest 'keep[ing] a record for a day or two of how your illness or disability affects you' (ibid.).

In focusing on singular behaviour, the state-sponsored model of disability promotes individual failing above any attention to environmental and social factors. The DLA pack rigidly constructs and controls the definitional parameters of what constitutes disability in such a way that those who need to place themselves within that definition are obliged to take personal responsibility in turning a critical gaze upon their own bodies. That the format of the DLA questionnaire was decided in consultation with disability rights groups merely reinforces the sense in which power/knowledge relies on self-surveillance. The claimant is

About help with personal

■ Part 2 Help you need – **during the day** – continued

■ **Coping with your toilet needs**

Roughly how many days a week do you need help

	No help needed	1 to 3 days	4 to 5 days	6 to 7 days
getting to the toilet?	☐	☐	☐	☐
using the toilet?	☐	☐	☐	☐
using something like a commode, bedpan or bottle instead of the toilet?	☐	☐	☐	☐
coping with incontinence of the bladder?	☐	☐	☐	☐
coping with incontinence of the bowel?	☐	☐	☐	☐
using a colostomy bag?	☐	☐	☐	☐
using incontinence aids, pads or nappies	☐	☐	☐	☐

How many times a day do you need help coping with your toilet needs?

Roughly how many minutes do you need help for each time?

Please tell us about any equipment that you use to help you with your toilet needs.
This could be rails by the toilet, a special toilet seat, or something like this.

Tell us as much as you can about the help you need coping with your toilet needs.
The more you can tell us, the easier it is for us to get a clear picture of the type of help you need.
For example, if you are a woman you may need help coping with your periods.

12

Figure 1.10 Page from *Disability Living Allowance* claims pack (1994), 'Coping with your toilet needs'. Courtesy the Benefits Agency

constrained to answer questions not just on her general capacity to negotiate successfully the everyday processes of washing, dressing, cooking and so on, but on the minutiae of functional capacity at every differential stage, and moreover at differential frequencies. Figure 1.10 (Section 2: 12) illustrates the extraordinary complexity and detail in which the claimant is expected to freely confess to her own bodily inadequacy. The questions for each discrete function follow a similar format, and many – like those on toilet needs – are duplicated to establish night-time behaviour as well. What this amounts to is an impressive display of power/knowledge, and of its capacity to proliferate discourse in accordance with Foucault's dictum: 'the exercise of power creates and causes to emerge new objects of knowledge and accumulates new bodies of information' (1980: 51). No area of bodily functioning escapes the requirement of total visibility, and further, the ever more detailed subdivision of bodily behaviour into a set of discontinuous functions speaks to a fetishistic fragmentation of the embodied person.

In a paper discussing the differential models of disability underlying patient-completed health status questionnaires, Ziebland *et al.* (1993) attempt to account for what they see as a not 'entirely rational accumulation' of assessment factors. The explanation lies, they claim, in the nature of information required to satisfy any one of four variant models; namely, the functional, subjective distress, comparative and dependence model. On a superficial level the DLA claim form might seem to draw heavily on the dependence and to some extent the functional model, but it remains difficult to account adequately for the depth of enquiry into the minute operations of the individual body. As the overt point of the allowance is to offset the unavoidable cost of help with everyday operations, it would seem that once a general category of need is established, nothing more is added by detailing precisely how often and which of the processes involved cannot be undertaken unaided. In the section on cooking a main meal, for example, the claimant is asked to distinguish between the inability to use a cooker and the inability to cope with hot pans (*DLA 580*, 1993: 16). Given the absence of any sufficient justification that could arise from the declared intentions of the welfare process itself, one must assume that the extent of the benefit agency's 'need' to know is indeed an expression of the power/knowledge complex that underwrites the modern social body. The welfare claimant, like Foucault's prisoner of the post-Enlightenment period, is controlled not by a display of external coercion but by continuous surveillance and by the insistent demand for a personal accounting. The subject herself effects a normalising judgment on her own modes of being, by submitting to what Foucault calls a power that 'produces domains of objects and rituals of truth' (1977a: 194). Moreover, my claim is that the one who acts is not a pre-existent bounded being, but that she constructs her very selfhood in the process of normalisation. In terms of the DLA claim form she produces herself as a disabled subject. What this display of the productivity of power signals is how control of the social body is effected through disciplinary technologies targeted on the individual body.

Where Foucault was concerned primarily to deconstruct the power relations between the singular, but universalised, body and a series of institutional structures – the prison, the clinic, the school – and to expose the symbiotic links between the individual disciplinary practices and the manipulation of population, feminists have been constrained to emphasise that those economies are gendered. The interplay of power and knowledge produces difference in just such a way that the bodies of women are the ground on which male hegemony and, at least in part, the power of the state in the service of capitalism are elaborated.[18] The polymorphous forms of domination to which we are subjected are frequently masked so as to appear freely chosen. Either they may appear expressive of personal desire, or they may be consented to as necessary for individual or social good. What is not always apparent, however, is that those goods and desires circulate within a system of normativities which, although never inevitable, impose nonetheless a powerful urge to behave in certain ways, to mark out the boundaries of the proper. Indeed the efficacy of disciplinary practices may be greatest when they appear not as external demands on the individual but as self-generated and self-policed behaviours. These internalised procedures constitute what Foucault calls the technologies of the self which

> permit individuals to effect, by their own means, a certain number of operations on their bodies, their own souls, their own thoughts, their own conduct, and this in a manner so

as to transform themselves, modify themselves, and to attain
a state of perfection, happiness, purity and supernatural power.
(1985a: 367)

In other words, the objectifying gaze of the human sciences which
fragments and divides the body against itself has its counterpart
in an insight which equally finds the body untrustworthy and in
need of governance. Moreover, each form of surveillance incites
the other.

In common with the disciplinary practices discussed above in
the context of an overseeing welfare state, the effect of such technologies is to render its subjects transparent. Whilst it is clear that
some groups of women, including those classed officially as
disabled, are marginalised by many of those operations which are
directed at 'whole' bodies, my point remains that all women are
positioned *vis-à-vis* an inaccessible body ideal. The particular
micro-politics of power which are worked upon the bodies of
women, and which are a focus of much recent feminist research,
take the forms of such commonplace occurrences as dieting and
weight control, elective cosmetic surgery, aerobics and body-
building regimes, and, as I shall later show in more detail, the
new reproductive technologies. The strategies of self-transforma-
tion extend, as Sandra Lee Bartky (1988) shows, from appearance
(clothes, make-up), through morphology ('figure') to comportment (expression and movement), and are apparently eagerly
taken up under the influence of ever new norms of behaviour. As
Bartky recognises, '[t]o subject oneself to the new disciplinary
power is to be up-to-date' (1988: 81). What is constructed here is
a constantly recirculated idealisation of femininity which requires
of its subjects an unremitting and impossible struggle to realise
perfection. Spitzack reports, for example, a failure rate of 98 per
cent among American women dieters (1987: 358).

The frustrated aspiration for the perfect body is not, it must be
stressed, a matter of inadequate will, but speaks instead to the
very nature of desire itself. Although the conception of desire
derived from Foucault is sometimes counterposed to that of Lacan,
for example, in that desire for the former is endlessly productive
while desire for the latter signals lack, I believe that the distinction misses the point of disciplinary power. In the Foucauldian
scenario such power generates desire, which, it seems to me, must
be productive in turn, precisely because it strives always to fill an
ever renewed lack. But what I want to suggest is that in any case

there is more involved than desire and lack. The reiteration of the technologies of power speak to a body that remains always in a state of pre-resolution, whose boundaries are never secured. Indeed, repetition indicates its own necessary failure to establish any stable body, let alone an ideal one. Moreover, the interchangeability of the practices of the self which operate within a logic of desire may remind us of the substitutability of hysterical symptoms as they elude always the closure of diagnostic knowledge. In alluding to the hysterisation of women's bodies as one focal point for regulatory control, Foucault may have evinced more than he intended. In the phallocentric order, the female body can never finally answer to the discursive requirements of femininity but remains caught in an endless cycle of bodily fetishisation that marks a failure of control.

The construction of what I take to be the illusion of docility, most fully realised in women where specific forms of domination attach to the material body itself, is established then not once and for all, but is sustained by continual procedures of both internal and external disciplinary power. Yet for all that these are technologies of control, the effect is not so much repressive as facilitating. Though women in contemporary society are always, but not only, inserted into the normativities of maternity, their bodies, as Linda Singer explains, must be multi-functional too, useful 'for wage labour, sex, reproduction, mothering, spectacle, exercise, or even invisibility as the situation demands' (1993, 'Bodies – pleasures – powers': 124). Rather than simply enforcing a restrictive sameness, as its position as one dominant element in the generation of normativities would seem to imply, the concern of health care with body management may appear to have a liberatory and individualising effect. As a result it makes little sense for feminism to cast health care and medical technologies as in any sense intrinsically inimical to women. This is much more than the simple observation that sometimes the intervention into bodies produces individual and social good. That much is clear, but my point here is that, given the inescapability of the relations of power, to say that they are necessarily bad is to say that everything is bad. Instead, like Foucault, I prefer the formulation that everything is dangerous; and particularly so when the microphysics of bio-power coalesce to support quasi-structural systems of domination such as the patriarchy – the very thing that Foucault tends to ignore.

Whilst by no means homogenous, many feminist critiques of health care have been, in any case, somewhat superficial, in that while some procedures are seen as wholly repressive, others – which in a Foucauldian analysis seem no less dangerous – are welcomed and even promoted as social ideals. The increasingly widespread use of ultrasound in pregnancy (now taken up by around 90 per cent of pregnant women), or triannual medical check-ups for the elderly are just two such examples. What a reading of Foucault suggests is that, first, bodies are not pre-given in some objective reality, but are specific, variable, and non-necessary historical and discursive constructions, and second, health care may be characterised not as disinterested beneficence or neutral scientific intervention, but as inextricably caught up in the technologies of power. It is a reading that must call into question the moral practice of the medical sciences. If there is neither a fixed reality of health and disease, nor yet a natural body to restore to good health, then what is at stake when health professionals intervene in the lives of individuals? Modern biomedicine, whether concerned with the single patient or with populations, is characterised by the strategies of normalisation which constantly measure, assess, record and project the limits of health. But far from being the 'sick' body which is at the centre of such surveillance, it is increasingly the case that the body in what is classed as good health must also submit to monitoring. It is not simply that various health promotion and preventive techniques targeted on the individual serve to reinforce arbitrary but normative dichotomies, but that the medical gaze oversees and constructs those poles in complicity with the subject herself. The institution, met with widespread feminist approval, of well-women clinics, for example, is hailed as an instance of women taking more control over their own bodies. Whatever gains that development may represent, however, it is nonetheless situated within a project of regulation through generalisation. Though there may be no technological fix, the operative discourse remains that within which bodies are not to be trusted nor differences acknowledged. The abnormal is to be rooted out, and recovered from its otherness by reincorporation into an ever expanding realm of the same.

In contrast, the excess that irrecoverably evades disciplinary power and the boundaries set in place by that power, the excess that resists and disrupts the strategies of identification, is both necessary to the establishment of normativity and the site of normative anxiety. And in a male-dominant social order, though Foucault has nothing to say directly of this, it is that which escapes femininity, the embodied but gender-resistant female subject, which provides the moment of contestation. The claim, it must be clear, is not that the bodies of women are ever outside the relations of power/knowledge, but that there is potential slippage between what is possible for them and what is required of them by even the most adaptive patriarchal state.

According to Foucault, modern power, unlike the sovereign/ juridical model which it has largely supplanted, is transformative of meanings and productive of truths, working on as much a discursive as a material level. Its relations are omnipresent, consti- tutive of 'reality' itself, so that there can be no position of exterior resistance as there would be to a unified and repressive force (1979: 95). The inescapability of power in a Foucauldian sense is quite different too from the notion of an all-pervasive ideology from which emancipation might be possible by comparing false consciousness with external truth. For Foucault there is no foun- dational truth, only other 'truths' which must arise within the relations of power itself. Accordingly, the notion of resistance is not that of a complementary but external force, but of multiple points of contestation generated by the very productivity of power itself. And though, as Foucault concedes, resistance may occa- sionally take the form of radical rupture, it is more usually local and specific:

> the points, knots, or focuses of resistance are spread over time and space at varying densities, at times mobilizing groups or individuals in a definitive way, inflaming certain points of the body, certain moments in life, certain types of behaviour.
>
> (Foucault 1979: 96)

Just as disciplinary power incites certain practices in which external expectations are internalised in forms of self-surveillance, so too those very same practices may ground resistance. Drawing on just such a site, Sawicki (1991: 64), for example, observes how certain female body-builders may exceed the feminine aesthetic and thus destabilise gender perceptions.

The absolute interconnectedness of power and resistance on which Foucault insists – '[t]here is no power without potential refusal or revolt' (1988: 84) – belies the accusation that his understanding of the production of docile bodies speaks only to passivity. But is the struggle ever a successful one, or rather what would constitute success amidst the relentless relations of power? Although Foucault speaks consistently of local and discontinuous points of resistance, there is no reason to suppose that they should not become, like the micro-practices of power itself, ever more extended and transformed by forms of global investment. What Foucault recommends is the recovery of 'disqualified, illegitimate knowledges' (1980: 83), which for feminists might point to the obscured histories of women and of their bodies. If it can be demonstrated that what has been naturalised as the truth of the female body is merely the discontinuous outcome of a complex series of normalisations, in which health care has been pre-eminently implicated, then it becomes possible to dissolve that devalued identity and theorise new constructions of female embodiment. Moreover, in contesting the universal signification of the living body we are obliged not to forfeit all knowledge of ourselves but to acknowledge the plurality of possible constructions and of the differences which exceed imposed normativities. There can be no one single locus of resistance, any more than there is a single locus of oppression, but that does not mean that there cannot be a legitimate, even collective project to disrupt the power of regulatory control and classification.

My account thus far makes no claims to give a continuous history of the body, but only to trace a series of relationships which consistently devalue female embodment. What the use of Foucauldian analytics exposes is that the nature of embodiment is defined with reference to the normative binaries of male/female, health/ill health, able-bodied/disabled, and so on. Contrary to the historically dominant discourses of bioscience, however, there is nothing determined about that embodiment: there are always counter-discourses, moments of resistance which undermine the stability of the naturalised and normalised model. Where Foucault spoke of self-imposed practices of the body, Judith Butler opens up new possibilities in her concept of performativity. She writes:

> acts, gestures, enactments, generally construed, are *performative* in the sense that the essence or identity that they otherwise purport to express are *fabrications* manufactured and sustained through corporeal signs and other discursive means. . . . This . . . suggests that if that reality is fabricated as an interior essence,

that very interiority is an effect and function of a decidedly public and social discourse.

(1990: 136)

What this proposes is that in performing our bodies in transgressive ways, we may subvert the apparent fixity of both raw
biological data and of our embodied selves. But what I want to
flag here is that the boundaries which organise us into definable
categories are in any case discursively unstable,[19] and it is not so
much that resistance is required to override them as constant reiteration is needed to secure them. Just as we perform our sexed
and gendered identities, and constantly police the boundaries
between sameness and difference, so too the purity of the healthy
body must be actively maintained and protected against its cont-
aminated others – disease, disability, lack of control, material and
ontological breakdown. In the context of embodied selves where
there is no distinction between mind and body, the claim to full
self-identity is still illusory. As Diana Fuss puts it: 'To the extent
that identity always contains the spector of non-identity within it,
the subject' (and I would stress here, in my similar move, the
embodied subject) 'is always divided and identity is always
purchased at the price of the exclusion of the Other, the repression or repudiation of non-identity' (1989: 102–3). To deconstruct
binary difference then, to point up all those oppositional categories which begin to undo themselves at the very moment of
defining identity through exclusion, disrupts both ontological and
corporeal security.

Interestingly, one strategy recently advocated in disablement
politics is to push the 'healthy' majority to a recognition that they
are merely temporarily able bodies. Although intended to mark
no more than the material precariousness of health, that slogan
can be extended to provide just that thoroughgoing critique of
health/ill health, able-bodied/disabled that a poststructuralist
approach would suggest. In other words, the regulatory and disciplinary regimes which impose and maintain normative standards
of bodily and mental well-being are necessary precisely because
of the inherent leakage and instability of categories, because the
spectre of the other always already lurks within the selfsame. What
a feminist project might aim to do is to uncover the mechanisms
of construction, flaunt the contradictions and transgressions which
destabilise the binaries, and insist on a diversity of provisional

bodily identifications. The move towards embodied selves need not entail a new form of essentialism nor a covert recuperation of biological determinism. Rather it celebrates embodiment as process, and speaks both to the refusal to split body and mind, and to the refusal to allow ourselves to be either normalised or pathologised. At the same time to stress both particularity *and* substantiality for the female body challenges the universalised male standard and opens up for us new possibilities of (well) being-in-the-world.

Chapter 2

Foundations

THE ETHICS OF MODERNITY

Having now indicated the discursive nature, not simply of what is taken to constitute health and disease, but of the body itself, I want to turn to the ethics that traditionally adheres to those constructions. Despite a recent history of often highly critical engagement with ethics, mainstream feminism has favoured recuperation of the major principles rather than deconstruction. In contrast, my own purpose is to offer finally a radical rewriting of what constitutes the ethical moment, but it is necessary first to trace an overview of what is at stake in the deconstruction of conventional systems. From the perspective of any feminist critique, it will quickly become apparent that the sexual difference which marks the modern body finds little overt expression in the foundational paradigms of modern ethics, nor yet in its derivative, bioethics. In addition, while a specifically female embodiment is unacknowledged, or worse, taken as the ground for disqualification from full moral agency, it is also the case that no body plays a material part in the dominant ethical systems. This is especially curious with regard to biomedical ethics.

Whatever else characterises it, health-care ethics is a morality directed towards bodily matters, and yet my claim is that for the most part it is itself disembodied, almost literally out of touch with lived experience. As a supposedly practical discipline what it purports to enquire into is largely the question of what should be done and by whom. Issues of agency are then central to its concerns; but though the turn is sometimes to singular embodied practices, the problematic is focused more often on conceptual generalities, such as the notion of consent. In any case, justificatory appeal is made to the universalised and abstract principles of the wider ethical theory which is built on a determined disavowal not only of the particularity of the sexed body, but of corporeality itself. The problem is not such that health-care ethics could or should be considered a distinct or detached field of enquiry, but that the paradigm moral theories on which it draws are themselves deeply flawed by their transcendental pretensions. Biomedical ethics is not a special case, but simply one area in which the tension between the material canvas on which moral action is played out, and the transcendental ground of justification, is highly uncertain. But more importantly, what I shall go on to argue in later chapters is not just that a conventional ethics is inappropriate to the concerns of health care, and marred by its indifference to the specificities of gender, race, class, sexuality and so on, but that the whole question of right and wrong, good and bad is fundamentally misconstrued. Before offering that more radical critique of foundational thinking, however, I shall outline some relevant issues and point up some inherent inconsistencies within the ethics of modernity.[1]

How, then, is moral agency established within the dominant discourse of Western ethics? The usual characterisation is as the realisation of the capacity to choose and act, freely and rationally, within a framework of moral requirements. Those demands require the agent to act on the calculations of some given utility; or in accordance with the rules of a pre-existing hypothetical contract with other members of the moral community; or according to the dictates of virtue. Of these doctrines the first two have been dominant in medical ethics and, though they may be mutually exclusive at the level of theory, in practice a substantive ethics such as that applied to the field of medicine is likely to be guided by some combination. And while there are other ways of conceiving moral agency which remain unaddressed by the major conventional paradigms – existentialism could stand as an example here – it will be my contention that all are predicated on certain necessary exclusions of which gender difference is a primary form. The feminist ethical project starts from the point that, far from being the gender-neutral pursuit of objective utilities or expression of intrinsic goods, as is claimed, morality is highly mediated by gender. This is not *necessarily* to deny that there are objective utilities or intrinsic goods, but to claim that if those are the central determinants of properly based moral reflection then the dominant discourse inevitably denies full moral agency to women. A brief look at consequentialism, most often expressed in its classical utilitarian form, and at deontology and related rights-based theories, which focus solely on those issues relevant to a feminist critique, will make this clearer.

The central claim of consequentialism that right action must be decided, not in accordance with some pre-existing set of values, but only by reference to the relative benefits and harms consequent on an intended action, is, of course, open to many objections. I shall say nothing of these, but note only that the theory demands that moral agency is firmly rooted in the exercise of a consistently calculative mentality, and that this in turn relies on some notion of rationality. In the absence of absolute rules of behaviour, each new set of circumstances potentially alters the parameters of good and bad action, and the individual must act on her own authority. It is important to note here that this apparent, and to some degree real, sensitivity to diversity nevertheless refers back to an actor who is not required to question her own position as arbiter. In other words, though the moral agent is continually engaged in, and responsible for, a series of finely tuned calculations which supposedly may be empirically verified, the apparently objective nature of the balancing act is necessarily underpinned by subjective judgments about the relative value of different benefits and harms. The ultimate failure of the attempt by consequentialist theories of moral action to strip away any trace of value judgments, and to present themselves as strictly rational and unbiased, is an important element in the deconstruction of traditional moral agency.

Despite the theoretical insistence that everyone, not excluding the agent, is to count as one only in terms of weighing up relevant interests, the undeniably overriding importance of the moral agent in consequentialism has important implications for women. In theory, the explicit prohibition on privileging the agent's own preferences above those of others supposedly guarantees the egalitarian nature of the exercise and ensures that the calculus has inter-subjective acceptance, or at very least acceptance amongst similarly rational persons. In effect, however, the agent remains in a uniquely powerful position, for in so far as value judgments are an inevitable part of the operation, then the initiating actor must rely on her own individual assessment of relative worth. Further, as she is committed to maximising the common good over and above any individual considerations, she is theoretically entitled, it seems, to override the interests of anyone who is not similarly willing – or deemed able – to make the appropriate calculation.

Now all this must call into question, on an abstract level, the egalitarian claims of consequentialism. More to the point, however, it is difficult see how, on a practical level, the system can avoid privileging the primary agent in any situation in which a power imbalance already exists. Given the social realities of male dominance, the problem for women must be particularly acute with regard to paternalism, which I define here as acting in someone else's supposed interests, but against her wishes and without her consent. The theoretical paternalism to which consequentialism lends itself all too easily translates into the very real paternalism exercised by men over women. In the medical encounter, in particular, the persistent imbalance between the sexes in terms of the professional role puts women at what turns out to be a philosophically legitimated disadvantage.

In response to a more general unease than specific gender considerations, many philosophers sympathetic to utilitarianism have tried to distinguish between hard and soft paternalism. Where the hard version would justify, even in the face of protest, action for someone else's own good if the moral actor believed it to maximise benefit, the soft version would formally prohibit intervention unless the other were not acting rationally. In other words, it would not be sufficient simply to substitute one's own values, or preferences, for those of another, however much they seemed to work in her favour, unless that person was either temporarily or permanently unable to make a rational assessment of her own interests. Taking up that proviso, Gerald Dworkin, for example, argues that certain paternalistic interference is to be seen as 'a kind of insurance policy which we take out against making decisions which are far-reaching, potentially dangerous and irreversible' (1976: 197). It is unclear, however, whether he believes simply that our rationality may be contingently compromised, or that by their very nature certain acts, like suicide, speak to an inherent irrationality. Less obviously contentious is the resort to paternalism as a rule of thumb in those medical encounters where the patient is unconscious, and yet there too its efficacy in maximising the patient's best interests is by no means certain. Imagine that one is unconscious and faced with imminent death unless given a life-saving operation. Providing there is no dispute about the acceptability of the quality of life which will ensue, the surgeon may legitimately assume that the patient would wish to be operated on. A small shift in emphasis, however, may make all the difference, for how is the surgeon to know in advance if the temporarily comatose patient – an accident victim, perhaps – would rather lose one eye now or risk blindness in both later? As it is difficult to claim decisively that either course would be more rational than the other, utilitarianism's much prized objectivity is once more compromised by a necessarily subjective judgment.

These are of course practical difficulties; but the ambiguity is no less evident on the abstract level. It is not simply that the intervention of a third party is problematic, but that it is not at all clear what a rational assessment of one's own interests might consist in. The question of the ideological construction of interests is scarcely considered, as though there were in fact some objectively recognisable goods. Similarly, the nature of rationality is taken to be transparent, and to devolve on a reductive argument: to act rationally is just to calculate the relative benefits and harms of one's intentions and to act in accordance with the greatest good. Even in its own terms then, appeal to a rational calculus often fails to provide a clear-cut guide for moral action, but is inextricably caught up in the agent's subjective judgments. And where acting on another's behalf is intended, what is assumed is the ability to assess nothing less than the other person's state of mind.

That an assessment of benefits and harms is intrinsic to health care is scarcely controversial, but the tendency to elide ethical utility with economic utility, in an overtly political form, results in an overdetermined reliance on utilitarianism as the primary system of justification. That is not to suggest, however, that there is a 'pure' ethics somehow untouched by socio-cultural considerations. The medical sociologist Nicholas Fox stresses just that point in his critique of the rationality model of late-twentieth-century British health care: 'However formalized the method of calculating ends, the underlying values by which these calculations come to have political significance determine the ethical engagement' (1993: 127). Nonetheless, Fox too seems unaware that the consequentialist approach is but one perspective in what might constitute a modernist ethics of health care. I shall turn to some alternatives shortly; but what concerns me primarily here is not so much the macro-level 'contamination' of the ethical, referred to by Fox, as the predication of the individual medical encounter on an almost inevitable imbalance of power. It is not just that the structural inequalities of race, class, gender and so on must mediate every encounter, but that at the simplest level the one – the patient – has a problem which the other – the health-care professional – might solve. What I am suggesting is that consequentialism grounds and legitimises the formal expression of that power relationship. While in cases of conflict hard paternalism makes no pretence of respecting the other's liberty to choose between options, the so-called soft version not only falls into making subjective value judgments about the weight of conflicting interests, but claims that it can measure the rationality of the thought process as well. Though it rejects the stark premise that 'the doctor always knows best' in favour of the option of saying that sometimes the patient doesn't know her own mind, it seems to me that the insidious operation of soft paternalism is every bit as disenabling to the patient. Certainly conscious motivation may be entirely well-meaning, but nevertheless its operation can impose unwanted conditions. It is, as Thomasma calls it, 'beneficence dumped on someone' (1992: 12). Either way, what paternalism does ultimately is to deny moral agency to the other. Moreover, as I shall show, the question of who is that other is a matter of primary importance.

As medical ethics becomes more widely accepted as a component in professional training, perhaps fewer doctors would expect to occupy, and fewer patients would be prepared to accept, the traditional conception of the role of the physician. Nonetheless, there are still out-and-out paternalists like Ingelfinger who, writing in arguably the most influential North American medical journal, was able to state: 'If you agree that the physician's primary function is to make the patient feel better, a certain amount of authoritarianism, paternalism and domination are the essence of the physician's effectiveness' (1980: 1507). This open-ended justification of professional dominance hardly accords with the utilitarian commitment that no party to a moral exchange may claim a priori privilege and that all relevant interests are to be taken into account. In so far as any doctor is professionally committed to providing the best possible care for a patient, it must be a minimal requirement that what is *medically* indicated is presented as one significant option; but that is hardly enough to decide the morally appropriate course of action. The issue is clearly more contentious where it may appear that the patient is indeed acting *without intent* against her own best interests, but nonetheless it is difficult to see what might justify a necessarily limited professional view of 'right' action. In general, however, the robust defiance of the principle of personal liberty seemingly advocated by Ingelfinger is masked by a concern to take the patients' wishes into account. Nonetheless, so long as the professional retains the option of side-stepping conflicting assessments of best interests by questioning the understanding or rationality of the patient, the encounter remains at best a one-sided moral exercise, rather than a negotiation between two equal moral agents. And while this must clearly affect all patients regardless of gender, I shall argue later that the woman patient's disadvantage is deepened not just by her psycho-social experience of sexism, but by the construction given to rationality itself.

In turning to ethical theories based around some form of hypothetical contract which binds together and regulates the moral community, the privileging of rationality as the basis of moral agency becomes if anything even more imperative. Though the contract may specify some goal of the common good which relies on a consequentialist moral field,[2] the major systems which work, either implicitly or explicitly, on the basis of contract are deontological. Leaving aside, as both less problematic for its adherents and less open to challenge from its opponents, those systems where the moral law represents a contract between some transcendental authority and the people, then the secular system proposed by Kant can be taken as representative. Indeed, it was his central contention that as individuals we give ourselves the moral law and 'discover' what it is through the exercise of rationality. What makes deontology attractive to the medical model is that it yields a clear set of duties which may serve as action guides to the providers, while at the same time pointing at the very least to concomitant rights which may protect the users of a medical service against the worst excesses of paternalism.

For Kant, the starting point of any conception of the moral universe was the notion of rationality, the attribute attached *potentially* to all persons by virtue of their common humanity. Whether he believed that women actually fell within this formulation is somewhat unclear, for although their humanity is allowed, full personhood seems to be denied. And it was persons who could by the exercise of reason alone arrive at what Kant termed the Moral Law which, as the wholly rational source of all duties, we are obliged to obey.[3] The basic principles of the law, unlike those of religious duty, were held to exist a priori and could be justified in solely human terms. By virtue of their rationality, all persons must, necessarily in Kant's terms, behave in certain ways demanded by what he termed the Categorical Imperative. The unitary basis of all subsequent duty-based morality was the condition that we should 'act only on that maxim whereby thou canst at the same time will that it should become a universal law' (Paton 1961: 67–8).

In the ideal situation, moral duty thus derived is straightforward and obligatory. It is not so much invented by human beings as simply, inevitably arrived at by pure reason; and while its discovery was through subjective reflection, its existence is an objective fact of human nature. Further, the corpus of duties is held to be the more objective, or at least inter-subjective, in being shared by all who are members of what Kant terms the moral community. The moral law, then, as the basis of the so-called original contract (the hypothetical agreement that makes social living possible) has the status of being binding, detached, unbiased and rational. Once in place it determines absolutely the parameters of moral agency and it is only by virtue of what Kant calls 'the sway of contrary inclinations' that transgressions occur. Nonetheless, for all the apparent inclusiveness of the self-given moral universe, Kant denied to women the right to speak for themselves, and thus, by implication, the ability to exercise reason in the categorical imperative. They are both *unmundig* (non-verbalising) and *übermundig* (over-verbal), and as such cannot fully attain the status of self-willed moral agents. It is not precisely that women are deemed incapable of developing their rationality, but that Kant believed that they should not be educated to do so. His repeated view was that 'laborious learning and painful pondering, even if a woman should greatly succeed in it, destroy the merits that are proper to the sex' (Kant 1981: 78). And those merits turn out to centre on her domestic capacity to act as the support of man. As Nancy Tuana points out (1992: 53), Kant clearly constructs the perfection of man as the end of humanity, and woman as a means to that perfection. And in first privileging rationality and then excluding women from full participation within it, he denied them the membership of the very moral community which would prohibit such means/end thinking.

Although Kantian deontology is not in itself rights-based, its powerful emphasis on rationality has more recently found favour with the contract theory proposed by Rawls (1972). In an attempt to suggest more clearly how we might arrive at the precepts of a moral community, Rawls has proposed a hypothetical scenario in which reasoning is conducted from behind a 'veil of ignorance' which denies to the individuals involved any extraneous knowledge of their own placement or of their real advantages and disadvantages in the world. It is Rawls's belief that, stripped of the knowledge necessary for personal partiality, we would mutually agree – by virtue of our common power of reason and inherent but non-specific self-interest – to adopt the principles of liberty and fair opportunity as basic rights. His assumption, like Kant's, is that the exercise of reason would inevitably lead to certain mutually acceptable conclusions, and further that each individual would at heart value an atomistic good, albeit expressed through common interests. Moreover, those principles of liberty and fair opportunity that supposedly satisfy the claims of justice and that generate the appropriate rights and duties which mediate the moral community are essentially centred on a supposedly gender-neutral and disembodied self.

As with most rights-based theories, the moral structure is then effectively competitive and individualistic, stressing the isolation of moral agents rather than their community. This emphasis is so highly characteristic of post-Enlightenment European philosophy that it needs to be flagged now that it is a contingent rather than necessary condition of moral agency. Although there are exceptions, particularly with regard to virtue-based morality, the more generally accepted model that is taken up in bioethics is of individually held rights which, to use Ronald Dworkin's word (1984), serve as 'trumps' against the demands of the common good. Similarly, one's duties are towards oneself and other individuals rather than to the community. In Western modernity the self is placed centre stage, and indeed autonomy, in the sense of independent self-determining individuality, is held as a self-evident good. That is not necessarily to claim, however, that self-determination is coincident with individualism. The emphasis on rights and duties which has evolved with the refinement of the liberal humanist discourse is not synonymous with Kantian deontology, and in any case in Kant's realm of ends, there would be no need for rights as such, as duty alone would bind each individual to act in a morally fair way towards all other members of the community. Autonomy was not here conceived as individualistic, but as a concept necessarily entailing respect for others as persons having their own ends. For Kant impartial respect was the essence of moral agency.

Although Kant's conception of duty implies no competitive field, it does nevertheless conjure up an image of human beings who, though universalised and undifferentiated in one sense, are also individually isolated in their moral decision-making. The reliance on abstract reason and the lack of contextual feeling allows for an ethics in which the demands of duty may be counter-intuitive within the specifics of a given situation. In consequence, the move from an abstract to an applied ethics, like bioethics, is highly problematic. And if rational reflection is taken to be the basis on which moral choices are made, then where conflicts arise between individuals they are likely to be resolved by the claim that one set of apparent duties is the result of imperfect reason. In a misapplication of Kant's theory the more powerful agent will simply privilege her own powers of reason. As with the utilitarian justification for medical paternalism, one could again be faced with the assertion that doctor knows best.

Post-Kantian deontology rarely takes specified duties as incontrovertible absolutes but relies on the relative flexibility of *prima facie* rules of behaviour which allow for resort to the notion of rights, not simply as the logical concomitant of duties, but again as some form of personal protection. The mere possession of rights, however, though clearly indicating membership of the moral community, does not mark the holder as a moral agent. The basis of a right may be either that it confers a specified inviolability – such as freedom or bodily integrity – which may not legitimately be interfered with; or that it entitles the holder to make certain claims on the services of others which they are obliged to give. The right to a decent minimum standard of health care might be just such a right. To hold a right, then, does no more than either prohibit or oblige action on the part of others; it does not seem to involve the holder in any moral activity. W may speak of exercising our rights, but that is distinct from simp holding them. A newborn baby, for example, may have a right t sustenance without that in any sense implying that a neonate is capable of moral agency. On the contrary, the holder of rights is somewhat at the mercy of the moral probity of others; and even the active user of rights does no more than exercise an entitlement. At most there is a *prima facie* assumption that her action would not be wrong. In short, a right confers an option, and as such is quite different from a duty which imposes a requirement, the enactment or denial of which constitutes the moment of moral agency. My point then is that although the two parties to a medical encounter may suppose themselves mutually participating in a moral contract, if the encounter is one based solely on professional duties and patient rights, then only one person – the practitioner – is engaged in moral agency.

THE ETHICS OF HEALTH CARE

In concentrating my remarks on utilitarianism and deontology, I do not mean to imply that those are necessarily the most important operative systems of moral thought in Western ethics. What I am claiming, however, is that where applied ethics is at issue – and this is particularly true for the field of bioethics – then the emphasis falls strongly, although rarely exclusively, on those two distinctive discourses which, moreover, are taken up in selective ways. Yet, as I have already outlined, each system has inherent difficulties which emerge even more clearly in the context of bioethics. So far the problematic has encompassed only those issues which arise if the normative and material framework are taken to be gender-neutral, and the concrete bodies on which an ethics is practised are themselves nonsexed. Once however the notion of sexual difference is introduced, it will be my contention that the relevant systems are not simply inadequate or inappropriate, but fundamentally untenable. For the interim, however, I shall approach the ethics of health care as though sexual difference were not an issue.

The formal discipline of biomedical ethics is, as I have already indicated, still very much at an early stage of development and could hardly have been said to exist as little as twenty-five years ago. Reflection on the moral responsibilities of health-care practice is very much older of course, as the Hippocratic Oath suggests, but it has been piecemeal and largely left to individuals to act according to their own cherished moral precepts. On a common-sense everyday level most of us would seek to resolve conflicts by appeal to and consideration of the notions of duty and utility, and in some senses the formal codes of recent years are scarcely more sophisticated. While, on the one hand, what might be called the 'principled' approach will draw on one normative system exclusively, regardless of the prescriptions it yields, on the other, the 'balance' approach may well combine those forms of moral reasoning which seem to answer best the needs of particular cases. More cynical commentators like Robert Holmes (1990) see this as arbitrarily choosing whichever theory best supports existing pre-critical or intuitive convictions on specific moral issues. No new moral insight is to be expected, and, as with the first option, appeal to meta-ethical justification does not come into play. Where Holmes sees this as evidence of an unbridged gap between bioethical problems and moral philosophy, Brody sees the same lack of theoretical unity as arising positively from the need to develop what he calls 'reflective equilibrium'. His claim, which exemplifies perhaps the course followed – though less critically – by many bioethicists, is that moral problem solving is a process whereby 'intuitions about particular cases may force us to revise our more theoretical beliefs, and this may lead to further revisions in our previously held beliefs about other particular cases. Nothing is final' (1990: 173).

The usual exposition of health-care or biomedical ethics tends, then, to take the form of listing certain principles which are taken as essential to good ethical practice, and whose local justification is drawn largely from a mixture of utilitarianism and deontology. What I am suggesting is that the field of morality in which biomedicine roots itself has tended to be a fairly restricted one in which the emphasis is firmly on those theories most likely to yield relatively clear guides to action. Nonetheless, certain concepts like formal justice, which in bioethics is usually understood as distributive justice, may yield different results according to which underlying theory is taken as primary. Although all may agree on justice as fairness, or more specifically as impartiality of treatment in the presumption of limited resources, the substantive criterium may be decided equally by utilitarian, egalitarian or libertarian theories. Most health-care practice tends towards a welfare model of justice based on needs, rather than on rights or deserts, for example, but, nonetheless, at the level of the individual encounter there may well be a conflict with the duty of care owed to the singular patient. That emphasis on care is not to be confused, however, with the notion of a relational, contextual care developed by the developmental psychologist Carol Gilligan (1982) and promoted by liberal feminist ethicists like Nel Noddings (1984) or Rita Manning (1992), but is on the contrary no less formal in its reliance on pre-given determinants than the appeal to justice. In conventional bioethics, the one towards whom we must act with justice or to whom an impartial duty of care is owed is the generalised rather than the concrete other (Benhabib 1986). The other and the self are both to be identified as contractors or agents within a rational moral system. What is called for in biomedicine is an instrumental ethics which will answer the limited question 'How should I act?', rather than a more nuanced consideration of the good as such, or of the other as distinct from the self.

Accordingly, it should always be borne in mind that my subsequent analysis of the inadequacy of conventional ethics engages with a similarly restricted range of discourses. That is not to say that the discourse of virtue ethics, for example, is ever entirely absent, and indeed it is increasingly heard in more recent analyses. In virtue ethics, the good resides not so much in what the moral agent does, but primarily in her being virtuous in herself. Rosalind Hursthouse's account of the ethics of reproductive care (1987, *Beginning Lives*), which explicitly takes a neo-Aristotelian approach, is one such example from the mainstream. Despite an evident sympathy to some feminist ends, Hursthouse's work stands clearly apart from a specifically feminist ethics of health care in which privileged notions such as caring are implicitly grounded in a reconstructed virtue ethics. Nonetheless, the predominantly problem-based approach of health-care ethics remains largely underwritten by utilitarianism and deontology. Amongst standard texts, for example, Beauchamp and Childress (1983) privilege autonomy, non-maleficence, beneficence and justice; Ranaan Gillon (1985, 1994) gives a similar list; Faulder (1985) adds veracity as a major principle; Downie and Calman (1987) give extra stress to autonomy and add utility; while Engelhardt (1986) grounds his libertarian approach on respect for individual autonomy, which he takes to be the fundamental condition of ethics itself. In contrast to these, Seedhouse (1988) seems to endorse a neo-Aristotelian ethic with his emphasis on health work as concerned with human flourishing and self-realisation (1988: 14), only to go on to produce an 'Ethical grid' (1988: chapter 9) to guide moral reasoning that clearly privileges deontological principles.

The implication throughout such texts is that health care is both part of the general field of morality, and that it forms a special area of concern, in that the relevant activity is itself pitched within a specific professional 'duty of care'. The idea is that doctors, for example, are like everyone else in being bound by certain moral precepts – such as telling the truth, keeping promises and so on – and that they are subject to additional constraints by virtue of their relationship with patients. The special duty of care, and indeed the fiduciary nature of the relationship, may find explicit expression in various professional codes of conduct, or it may remain at an implicit quasi-contractual level. The whole emphasis of the works cited, and of many others, is that it is the part of the doctor and other professionals to set the moral content of the encounter. With few exceptions,[4] the assumption seems to be that the provider is the primary or sole moral agent and that the most the user can do is to stake out her rights. In an extension of the general schema, Seedhouse (1988: 130–2) places the principle of creating and respecting autonomy centre stage. Nonetheless, although partially successful in shifting the emphasis away from professional self-concern, his formula still leaves intact the image of the provider as the sole agent. In endeavouring to both create autonomy in and enact respect for the existent autonomy of the patient, the professional may be forced to acknowledge the other as a potential actor in her own right, but in the specific encounter the moral economy is still largely one-sided. What Seedhouse has in mind here, and in his earlier model which positions the removal of obstacles to achievement as the central priority (1986: 61), is that health care should be an enabling exercise with patient self-determination as a desirable end. What is not considered is that self-determination might equally be seen as a desirable means; for although he privileges respect for autonomy, it is in the sense of not overriding the patient's own choices, rather than in the sense of joining with the patient in sharing responsibility.

What I am suggesting is that the injunction to respect autonomy can simply act as a prohibition or limit on certain actions rather than as a positive move to embrace the interests of the other in mutual determination. Moreover, the sense in which the professional implicitly remains the primary moral agent in the Seedhouse scenario is further emphasised by the principle of creating autonomy. It is not clear that it is within anyone's power to 'create' autonomy for another (though clearly removing obstacles is a necessary precondition), nor if it were possible would the moral hegemony of the doctor be challenged. The commitment to create, and arguably too to respect, autonomy must surely be highly individualistic, rather than a co-operative venture. Moreover, though *ethicists* are acutely aware at least of the moral relationship – though more rarely of the power relationship – between the providers and users of health care, some *practitioners* may hardly see the transaction as involving a mutual relationship at all.

This emphasis on an atomistic morality speaks to a highly dualistic way of representing reality which is characteristic of Western ontology and epistemology. And of course those dominant concerns are reflected not just in ethical systems as I have argued, but also in the very way in which human bodies are discursively constructed. In the first place, the major traditional model of health care, the so-called medical model, is saturated with dichotomies such as mind and body, science and nature, health and disease. Further, as I have already shown in the preceding chapter, the meaning and 'truth' of male and female bodies has been differentially figured to serve as the ground for the devaluation of women by men. And in terms of the ethics of health care, that gender devaluation is deeply implicated in and interwoven with the imbalance of moral agency in the doctor–patient dyad which itself expresses a typically dichotomous focus of concern.

Once the distinction, central to modernist biomedicine, between the healthy and diseased state is taken as self-evident, the supposition is that health care has the teleological purpose of defeating disease and treating clinical disorder. Where Foucault could characterise classical medicine and ethics as closely linked in the care of the self, the advent of modern science has encouraged the treatment of human beings as primarily abstract and malfunctioning machines, which has in turn the effect of strictly limiting the moral concerns of the doctor. By pathologising individuals and positioning them as objects of the clinical gaze, the health care professions have silenced the voice of the patient. Rather than being concerned with the lived body of socially situated individuals, traditional medical practice implicitly bases itself on the standard of an objective, universalised body. At worst, there is no need to see the other as a moral agent in any sense at all, let alone as an equal one, and it is therefore sufficient that she be treated with technical proficiency rather than with care and concern. Indeed, the basic principle of medical practice has been 'primum non nocere' ('first, do no harm') rather than the more positive injunction to beneficence, but either way the implication is that so long as the physician discharges her own strictly medical duty, then there is unlikely to be any ethical problem. The apparent conflation of medical with moral satisfaction underlies the more sophisticated question of the parameters of moral agency.

Now, although the restoration of a person to a medically normative state does not formally entail an ethical dimension, it remains the case that in practice the majority of doctors do in fact recognise that intervention – even in terms of the medical model – is just a matter of moral concern. Most modern professional codes of conduct reflect this, as does the Hippocratic Oath itself. Doctors are enjoined to cast themselves in a moral relationship with their patients, but this entails no more than that they should recognise and discharge their moral duties towards the essentially passive other. Yet there is no more sense of mutual moral agency in this than there is in my belief that I should not cause unnecessary suffering to my cat. I may grant that my cat has certain rights to well-being, but it makes no sense to imagine that she is in any way a moral agent. And so it is with traditional medical practice. The patient may be objectified as the passive recipient of professional medical, and hopefully moral, concern, but accorded no moral status in her own right.

And while a highly medicalised health-care service remains the dominant sphere of activity, then the underlying assumption of the duality of health and disease ensures that the patient's own interests may in any case seem largely irrelevant. Any doctor working within the conventional model, and having, as the result of extensive training and experience, expert and specific knowledge of disease processes, is encouraged to give help and advice on a narrowly reductionist level focused on illness and disease. What may be missing is any concern for what might be the patient's own, quite reasonable, wish to assess her choices in a much wider context. The strict medical model, even where it does encompass moral endeavour, simply has no place for the more extensive considerations – such as the effect of treatment on work or family life, for example – which an individual patient will think important. My point is graphically illustrated in an article by Martha Swartz, an American lawyer working in the field of institutional medical law. She records the responses of a group of predominantly male obstetricians to a hypothetical case in which a young and financially insecure pregnant woman refuses to remain in hospital for intravenous therapy to stop premature contractions. The woman argues that she needs to go home to care for her existing 2-year-old child for whom she is unable to make alternative arrangements. Swartz continues:

> [t]he majority of physicians present advocated petitioning the court for an order compelling the patient to stay in the hospital to avoid a premature delivery. They viewed the patient as 'hysterical' and were unsympathetic to her childcare needs. Few had any compunctions about physically restraining the patient should she refuse to voluntarily abide by the court order; they saw no distinction between this *competent* pregnant woman's refusal of treatment and an *incompetent* patient's noncooperation with treatment.
>
> (1992: 53)

It is not simply, then, that the patient is being denied the opportunity of independent moral agency, but that a necessary sensitivity to the parameters of moral concern is missing. Moreover, even if medical encounters were only simple technical exercises (though it is difficult to say when in fact they are only that), superior professional expertise should not be assumed. Several sociological studies of, for example, the medical management of pregnancy detail instances in which professionals deny women's own expertise and seek to reduce pregnancy to just another illness (Oakley 1980; Graham and Oakley 1986). The women studied were frequently ignored, patronised or deliberately confused in those instances where their own observations did not accord with the doctor's expectations. The desire to reduce reproduction to a scientific basis firmly under professional control represents a clear case of trusting only what can be measured and tested, at the expense of feeling, intuition and subjective lay experience. The women concerned were effectively denied both medical and moral access to the course of their own pregnancies.

Now clearly the functioning of such an imbalanced relationship is related to the pre-existing relations of power which mediate any encounter between the provider and receiver of health care.[5]

It is not just, as Beauchamp and Childress put it, that 'in clinical medicine patients are often abnormally weak, dependent and surrender-prone' (1983: 89), nor even that that vulnerability puts patients at a disadvantage with respect to both need and relative power. Rather, I would suggest, their powerlessness in the clinical situation is due in part only to any illness they may be experiencing. Whatever the particular practice of any individual doctor – and obviously very many are committed to a somewhat less authoritarian relationship with their patients – the general moral self-centredness of the role is reinforced by a discourse which always already privileges the attributes commonly associated with the provider. In its operations on both a real and ideal level, the dominant medical discourse – itself part of a wider episteme of binary oppositions – serves to establish, justify and perpetuate the inequality of the medical encounter. Where on the professional side are supposed to lie the standards of reason, scientific expertise, objectivity and authority, on the side of the patient are passion, intuition, personal experience and dependency. For the moment I shall do no more than flag the fact that those two sets of diametrically different attributes correspond, by and large, to the stereotypes of respectively male and female personality; and to note further that women under patriarchy are persistently disempowered in relation to men. My point here is that given the positioning of medical discourse within the Western intellectual tradition which overwhelmingly privileges the rational standard, it is small wonder that the mediating voice of medical practice is that of paternalism.

AUTONOMY AND CONSENT

What a conventional critique of health-care practice, and particularly that centred on the medical model, intends is to reform, rather than reconstruct, a set of given principles so as to provide a more egalitarian praxis. The emphasis remains firmly within the remit of liberal humanism and would thus cover a number of liberal feminist approaches, including, for example, Carolyn Faulder's *Whose Body is It?* (1985), and the more implicitly ethical approach of handbooks like *Our Bodies, Ourselves* by the Boston Women's Health Book Collective (1976; revised British edition 1978). If, as seems apparent, health-care users are not best served in a moral sense by the traditional concentration on non-maleficence and beneficence (both of which inevitably centre moral agency on the professional), then other strands of morality need to be given increased emphasis. Instead of simply taking the capacity for self-determination on the side of the professionals as a given, but as of little relevance for users, many current theorists of medical ethics, as already outlined, place autonomy centre stage. The autonomy of the doctor is as ever assumed, but new impetus is given to the belief that good ethical practice will enhance, or at least respect, the autonomy of the other in any medical encounter.

Both deontologists and utilitarians alike can see value in such a manoeuvre;[6] and, of course, the free-choosing individual is at the heart of an existentialist ethics. The drawback, as I have already indicated, is that even the radical step further advocated by Seedhouse (1988) of actually seeking to create autonomy does not fundamentally dethrone the dualism between provider and user which is not simply neutrally descriptive, but which always privileges the former. Nonetheless, given that autonomy is conventionally recognised as a determining feature of moral agency, the theoretical extension of it to both sides of an encounter would seem to indicate the potential for joint agency. Instead of expressing the traditional practitioner–patient dyad in terms of a subject–object relationship, the move is towards conceptualising both participants as potentially self-actualising subjects. The relatively recent and growing emphasis given to counselling as an integral feature of primary health care represents on the surface at least a conscious attempt to render audible the voice of the patient and to extend her sense of subjectivity and agency. But as the medical sociologist Carl May points out, though the health-care encounter is recast as mutually determined, the intended outcome remains one of patient compliance. And, as he puts it: 'Such interactions can have the effect of symbolically reconstructing highly problematic *structural* situations, and thus engender docility rather than agency' (May 1993: 9). This would seem to imply that the freedom of the patient participant remains severely restricted by existing power differentials. May makes no attempt to specify which structural factors he has in mind, but, as I shall go on to argue, the determinant of gender must surely be one of them.

In fact, the furthest that progressive liberal humanist theory seems able to go in reforming itself is to construct a model in which supposedly gender-neutral individuals meet together, as co-active and putatively equal moral agents, in a relationship mediated by a complex series of rights and duties. And though that may certainly represent a greater ethical sophistication than older models, its usefulness is strictly limited. In any case, though I would concede that some degree of self-determination is indeed a necessary, though not (always) sufficient, feature of moral agency, the liberal humanist concept of autonomy is at best a restricted form of self-determination. And moreover, as I shall argue, that particular formulation is at root incompatible with the feminist requirement that moral agency should extend to women. Even where the concept of autonomy is taken in its own gender-indifferent terms, and its suppression or promotion in prac-tice is seen to underlie the whole relationship between providers and users, it is, nonetheless, an autonomy which is manifest most often in a highly reductive way. The issue of consent is at the forefront of bioethical analysis, and is rightly of high moral concern in liberal theory, but too often it marks the limit of patient self-determination. I want briefly here to look at the parameters of consent as it is presently conceived, and to note that despite the assumption of gender neutrality it is especially problematic for women.

The issue revolves round two seemingly disparate loci: first, the notion of what it is to be a moral agent at all, which devolves on questions of subjectivity; and second – and this is particularly relevant to health care – what relationship exists between the 'I' who makes choices, who consents, and the body of that agent. Clearly any critique of consent which takes health care as its substantive field must inevitably come up against the materiality of the body, and what is interesting is the way in which women are both more clearly identified with their bodies, and are paradoxically denied the capacity to exercise moral agency over their own bodies. As I outlined in the first chapter, women are supposedly rooted in base corporeality, positioned, as Sartre would have it, in themselves, *en soi*, rather than for themselves, *pour soi*. And it is this supposed immanence that provides the justification, within the discourse of liberal humanism, for the exclusion of women from the attribute of full rationality, which is one of the essential parameters of moral agency. As a consequence, women are denied control of the very bodies which they have failed to transcend. More will be said of this in the following chapters.

How then does consent figure in conventional health-care ethics? Perhaps it needs to be flagged again that in so far as such an ethics has existed at all until quite recently, consent was one feature that was conspicuously absent from its field of enquiry. The proper conduct of medicine, and by extension more widely health care, required no more than that the professional should act in accordance with the dictates of either duty or utility: the first of which provides little scope for patient participation; while the other has notoriously lent itself to the very worst excesses of nonconsensual treatment. The claim of benign paternalism has until very recently been used to justify gross forms of interference with the human body, while the duty of beneficence continues to underwrite equally intrusive procedures. The hotly debated issue of unconsented caesarian sections illustrates the extended scope of the latter consideration, for there need be no claim that action is taken for the direct benefit of the patient, but may devolve solely on doing good to the as yet unborn foetus (Callahan and Knight 1992; Swartz 1992; Draper 1993). In practice, the liberal ideal of moral equality has tended at best to mean no more than a reductive focus on the issue of patient rights, but even the supposedly fundamental 'natural' right to bodily self-determination turns out to give strictly limited protection to the patient. Moreover, where the boundaries between self and other, on which the dominant ethics relies, are themselves indistinct – as in pregnancy – then the appeal to models of moral autonomy are inevitably strained.

What then constitutes consent in its normative sense? While everyday usage does habitually point to a simple 'agreement to' as its basis, a more rigorous approach quickly establishes the notion that a valid consent must be based on certain predetermined criteria concerning both the context and the status of the agent. These conditions turn out to be closely related to the criteria for autonomy itself, although the former may be more flexible. First and foremost, the consenter must be neither coerced nor intimidated, but free to make an autonomous choice. Second, the person must be both capable of consenting, which means in effect at least minimally rational, and in possession of sufficient relevant information about what is at stake. It makes no sense to say, then, that a person has consented unless she is free from (external) pressure and is able rationally to consider the options. Accordingly, we are reluctant to attribute the ability to consent, except for the most trivial cases, to all those – be they the very young, the senile, the learning impaired, the incarcerated – whose freedom or rationality is limited. What remains is a whole corpus of persons, both male and female, of all ages and varying degrees of health, who – at least, theoretically, within liberal humanist discourse – are equally entitled to be treated as responsible moral agents exercising their option of consent. Nevertheless, this ideal construction is deeply problematic on a linked series of levels, material and discursive, not least of which is that of sexual difference.

Although my own major focus throughout is on sexual difference, I want, always, to avoid the implication that there is any universal key to the structuration of power. The variables are never less than multiple and complex; and moreover, although the majority of, and perhaps all, women may be subjected to some forms of male-identified power, it is clearly not the case that all suffer equally or in the same way. The issue of obstetrical intervention is again instructive. In one Canadian study of a range of court-ordered interventions involving Caesarian sections, hospital detentions, and intra-uterine transfusions, it was found that 51 per cent of the women involved were non-white, 44 per cent were unmarried, and none were privately funded, from which we may infer that all were welfare recipients (Kolder *et al.* 1987). It is clear that although the threat of unconsented intervention hangs over all reproductively active women, in practice its operation is overdetermined with respect to particular women. A similar complexity extends beyond the concrete manifestations of power to its discursive exclusions of not just the female, but an irreducible diversity of what we may term 'other others'. The feminist project of exploiting the contradictions and tensions within the logos may concentrate – as I suggested in Chapter 1 – on recuperating the embodied feminine, but its implications extend to all those who fall outside normative paradigms.

In terms of Western health care the medico-ethical construction of what is meant by consent is mirrored and enforced by legal discourse. It is not the case that morality and the law are necessarily coincident; but, in a liberal democracy, they are rather more than merely coextensive. And given that in any case ethical paradigms are discursively constructed, not discovered, it is instructive to review other aspects of the power/knowledge nexus that constitutes authoritative discourse. It is worth noting that the currently seminal text of English medical law (Kennedy and Grubb 1994) devotes a total of over 300 pages to the issue of consent, much of which is taken up with the question of who is entitled to give it. The general criteria are those, first, of competency, which usually means being of a sound, rational, adult mind, and, second, of freedom from external constraint. The areas of teenage consent, the competency of psychiatric patients, or the validity of consent given by prisoners are matters of especial concern. Nowhere, however, does sexual difference appear as a variable, except in very specific instances, generally to do with issues of reproduction. Abortion and surrogacy, for example, self-evidently involve the consent of women; but in legal terms that is purely accidental. Thus, the *criteria* for male and female consent are the same.

As one major strand within the dominant discourse of liberal humanism, and as one which is held to reflect moral norms, the law must present itself, above all, as neutral, impartial and objective. Its proper concern is with the discharge of abstract contracts made between formally equal individuals involving, in health care as elsewhere, a network of mediating duties and rights. The real, embodied, *gendered* individuals who are in practice its concern, are, for the purposes of jurisprudence, held to have no legally significant differences – save the ones already mentioned – which affect the parameters for the categories of those who can and those who cannot consent. What is clearly missing from this picture is any notion of differential power, which, as a poststructuralist critique will make clear, operates on both a material and discursive level. In Chapter 1, I showed how a reading of Foucault would exemplify the way in which the modern social and political forms of liberal humanism position bodies – and in so far as Western liberal humanism is coextensive with patriarchy, they are women's bodies – as the location of regulatory power. And further, I shall go on to show that while an Irigarayan perspective should alert us to the violent exclusion of women from moral discourse, a Derridean deconstruction of the Western logos will problematise the very notion of consent, indeed of moral agency itself. But before that poststructuralist critique is employed, I shall focus on the dis-ease that is readily apparent within the common discourse of medicine and the law.

On a non-contentious level it is simply a matter of empirical observation that Western laws are formulated by an almost exclusively male legislature, and applied and interpreted by an equally male-dominated judiciary – in other words, by those whose experience of consent is situated on the side of power. And in so far as the law does concern itself with consent, it is as an essentially reactive concept. There is little or no interface with proactive choice, still less with notions of desire. The point is to offer protection from something rather than enabling the one who consents to do something. As far as health care is concerned, the legal notion of consent as a limit on the actions of others reinforces the intrinsically passive nature of patient 'participation'. But aside from mirroring the existing power differentials of health care, medical law goes further in compromising the option of consent. My point is that although patient self-determination is often referred to as a basic legal right,[7] its certainty is undermined not just by the claims of conflicting rights and duties, but also by the discursive exclusions of rationality. Where disputes arise – which usually involve negligent treatment rather than actual assault on the body – the standard set for a legally valid consent devolves on what a reasonable doctor is entitled to do, and obliged to divulge, in keeping with the current standards of her speciality, rather than on what a reasonable patient might choose for herself were she in possession of all the relevant information. In other words, the notion of a fully informed consent relies currently not on the patient's own subjective interests but on what the reasonable (and one might add potentially paternalistic) doctor would judge them to be.[8] The assumption would seem to be that only disinterested rationality is to count fully and that only the professionals are capable of exercising it. It is a case of both privileging rationality and denying it to certain specific groups. For women, that disempowerment is compounded in that in a society based on normative male standards they are not considered fully rational in the first place.

Nor are women any more able to fulfil the other criterion for the exercise of a valid consent; namely, in being free from pressure. Where men's interests conflict with those of women, that freedom is self-evidently lacking. An agreement to sexual intercourse, for example, given by the woman who is mentally, rather than physically, coerced would by no means fit a legal definition of non-consensual sex, yet surely it cannot be said to exemplify freedom of choice. The dominant material, physical and psychological power of men over women is simply unacknowledged in the fiction that the transaction is between two equal moral agents. The woman's interests are simply overturned by her own prudence if not by actual threat of future violent sanctions. But more invidiously, it may well be argued that even where consent is freely given, in the sense that the woman apparently shares the interests of the man, those interests are constructed within a power/knowledge complex which privileges men. It is not that women are necessarily victims of men, but that in patriarchal society they are disenabled by those discursive and non-conscious strategies of power which construct them as morally inferior.

So, what exactly does the term 'autonomy' – taken above as the implicit ground for consent – mean when used in the context of general ethics? I take it that far more is intended than the simple denotation of independent being, for though it may make some sense to speak of a newborn baby as an autonomous individual, we do not mean that she has the here-and-now capability of exercising autonomy in the moral sense. As with consent, the two features in which moral autonomy is grounded are freedom and rationality, and it is these which are problematic for feminism. In so far as the critique I shall offer occupies the familiar ground of liberal humanism, it might be argued in part-response that the notion of autonomy is at best an ideal, fully realisable only in some equivalent of Kant's realm of ends, and that for the purposes of applied philosophy what matters is the process. That is true; but if the ideal represents some hypothetical improvement against which that reality can be measured, then it is clear that one is entitled to contest the ideal. The argument is both that the concept of a universally applicable autonomy is untenable in both the social and moral sense; and that even were that not so – that there were no unbridgeable gap between real and ideal – then it has in any case little useful meaning in morality. That structure of argument in the alternative is precisely the mark of liberal feminism, but my account will go much further to deconstruct the very epistemology and ontology on which moral concepts are grounded. First, however, I shall continue to uncover the tensions already inherent to the notion of autonomy.

At first, the initial condition of autonomy, that of freedom for the individual, seems unproblematic. We understand it to mean both passive freedom from interference and active freedom to do something. In theory the agent must be neither coerced nor constrained by external forces, and she must have the capacity both to conceptualise and act on, though not necessarily achieve, the relevant desire. In other words, real choices must be accessible and must be made, for it would make no sense to suppose that the individual showed autonomy in simply following a predetermined course in life. But the notion of freedom rapidly runs into difficulty unless we further distinguish between the state of having the will to act autonomously and the actual exercise of autonomy. The latter, I take it, is unproblematic and fits the conditions already outlined; but what of the former? Can we speak meaningfully of individual autonomy where the person concerned is in fact restrained in her actions? It may be that she is perfectly capable of action were it not for some pre-existing restriction. A paraplegic, for example, may well think it right to visit her ageing aunt in hospital and may clearly want to do so, but if her disability prevents it are we then to deny her autonomy? In the social sense of exercising her choices, it is true, the autonomy of the woman is compromised; but in another way the very capacity to formulate choices and to distinguish preferences indicates an autonomous will and perhaps that is sufficient for what might be termed moral autonomy. The issue is clearer if we consider a prisoner of conscience, for it would be simply counter-intuitive to imagine that someone incarcerated for the expression of a strongly held moral belief could then be considered to lack moral autonomy. What seems to be important in both cases is the capacity to reflect on choices rather than a thoroughgoing freedom to act. But important though that concession may be, indeed crucial to the notion of autonomy as process, it has a significant drawback: it rests on the as yet unchallenged assumption of that capacity to choose as though it were some given of the human condition. Further, although the 'mental' autonomy described may satisfy a necessary condition, it can no longer be posited as a sufficient condition of moral *agency*.

It is the second fundamental ground of moral autonomy, rationality – that is, the capacity to reason and think logically, to choose desirable and effective ends – that is somewhat more disputed. A counter-tradition, exemplified by Hume,[9] makes man the slave of passion, and that the ground of an autonomous will; but nonetheless the dominant ethical paradigm, and certainly the one most influencing contemporary biomedical ethics, privileges rationality. Autonomy, then, is generally limited to those persons of sufficient age, experience and mental stability that their thought processes would stand up to logical scrutiny. It is worth noting that, for what might be termed social autonomy, the attribute of rationality is a desirable though optional extra, for no one supposes that those who act on irrational or badly reasoned premises are not self-directed. The category of *moral* autonomy, however, is ascribed only to those who are able to construct, think through and understand the nature of their choices. This goes much further, note, than simple consent which devolves on a set of predetermined choices which may have been made by another. Those in various categories of immaturity, mental disorder, to some extent physical sickness, and so on are not considered morally autonomous to the extent that they are not held responsible for their actions. And as with the condition of freedom the issue of access to choice is crucial, for true rationality must consist in the ability to distinguish between alternatives on a logical basis.

The major difficulty arises as to how to characterise the autonomy of those whose capacity to think and reason logically is unquestioned, but whose access to alternatives is limited by what may well be an unperceived restriction to certain modes of thought. This is exemplified by the individual slave, potentially *morally* autonomous by virtue of her humanity, but indoctrinated to the point of being unaware of such freedom. Yet it is an issue not only *in extremis*. As Judith Butler observes in another context, we are all constrained by 'not only what is difficult to imagine, but what remains radically unthinkable' (1993: 94). Freedom and rationality are both compromised by non-conscious ideological constraints which operate to make us incapable of knowing that even our thought processes are socially constructed rather than self-given. In such a case the ascription of autonomy seems inappropriate. The classic philosophical manoeuvre to escape this dilemma – which might be taken as paradigmatic for women under patriarchy – constructs something along the lines of:

> *A* would have the capacity (for autonomy) were it not for condition *X*.

This may theoretically satisfy, but in side-stepping all empirical grounding, the resultant formula tells us nothing of the actual material conditions of autonomy. It fails to confront the issue of power, for example, which determines not simply who can exercise autonomy, but even who shall have the capacity for its basic abstract requirements. If applied philosophy is to offer any realistic guidance then it cannot afford to retreat into arid analytic abstractions.

Now, although I have distinguished between moral and social autonomy, it remains the case that individual autonomy in a social context just is a matter of moral concern. It is not as though there were some abstract sphere of morality and another empirical state of society, for it is surely in the very positioning of an individual in a social context that she becomes a moral agent. Where behaviour falls entirely outside an inter-personal context, then it is doubtful that it could be deemed moral any more than it could be deemed social, though at the limit, as solitary individuals, we might behave towards ourselves in a more or less moral way. Nonetheless, our more usual understanding demands at the very least that our moral behaviour is directed towards other sentient beings, and I shall insist that it is primarily in the context where those beings may themselves be agents, that we are fully morally engaged. In any other context the exercise of autonomy is stripped of meaning and value, and consequently one can claim that it is only the socially situated individual who may be fully self-determined in any important sense. What counts in this linking of the social and the moral is that the choices to be made and the will to act reflect on an inter-subjective reality.

It is instructive to note here that where the ideal of autonomy has been most strongly championed in health-care ethics, it has given support to a libertarian perspective. On the one hand, the autonomy of practitioners has been fiercely defended against state interference, while on the other, that of users has been promoted as the requirement to respect patient choice. In both cases the individualistic ideal comes up against the reality of – amongst other things – scarce resources which must signal at some level a demand for mutually agreed limits which promote a common good. What such strains throw into focus is the general question of whether the notion of individual autonomy is fully compatible with self-determination as socially contextual, and that in turn has important implications for the further consideration of the efficacy of autonomy as the basis of moral agency.

In summary, then, the notion of moral agency most widely associated with modern thought positions it as the potential or actual province of all human beings who have the capacity for autonomy, who understand themselves to be bound by rights and duties, and who know themselves to be individuated subjective beings. In that formulation the issue has been addressed as though it were neutral and objective, an ahistorical concept, applicable to all relevant persons at all times in history. But though some of the internal strains and potential inadequacies of that discourse have been outlined, its epistemic and ontological centrality has yet to be challenged. In acknowledging the inevitably social basis of moral agency the ground is set to adopt a fully constructivist perspective which would view modernist ethics as no more than a specific construct, historically centred in post-Enlightenment Western philosophy.

Chapter 3

Fractures

THE CRITIQUE OF MODERNITY

My purpose in this chapter is to go on to critique in more detail both the general privileging of rationality – on which autonomy relies – and the appeal to closed and homogeneous categories. In particular, the supposed gender neutrality of the universal subject of mainstream Western philosophy – which is taken up uncritically in bioethics – will be exposed, not simply as masking gender privilege, but as a necessary feature of the modern episteme. The question arises as to why and how that particular discourse has been successfully positioned as the 'right' or 'true' one, and who its agents must necessarily be. What I am suggesting is that ethics, and indeed all philosophy, must be read textually as performing the very strategies of closure and exclusion which make truth claims possible, but which are taken as categories of the real. Moreover, what may appear to be no more than a contingent and political exclusion of women turns out to be a move that cannot be reformed, for it lies within a system which is founded on the very principle of exclusion. If women are to be valorised, then the paradigms of modernity must be subjected to a process of radical deconstruction. On the simplest level, as a reading of comparative philosophy should begin to show, any number of systems may offer alternative views of moral agency, and it is as well to remember that modern Western philosophy, though it lays claim to universal applicability, does not exhaust all forms of epistemology, ontology and ultimately ethics. For the present, however, it is enough to show that the Western tradition itself is far from unitary in its understanding of the essentials of moral personhood and moral agency.

What I have referred to as the modern period of Western philosophy dates from the mid-seventeenth century when what Kuhn (1970) would call a 'paradigm shift' occurred in the way we view ourselves as persons. For reasons which cannot be detailed here, but which undoubtedly relate to that whole nexus of inter-contextual exploration of both the classical past and the limits of contemporary knowledge, the individual, the subjective self, became paramount. The initial step of resolution of Cartesian doubt – the *cogito* – marks the self, the individual, as the primary actor at the centre of his own universe. And the new ontology inevitably generated a new ethics, such that Kant, for example, while believing dispassionately in the authority of god, was at pains nonetheless to construct a moral system independent of that transcendental *imprimatur*, and based instead on self-authorised agency. In Kantian ethics, which I take as paradigmatic of modernism and a major influence on conventional theories of bioethics, moral agency is a matter of the individual will which must necessarily choose to follow the dictates of duty, not because god has ordained it, but because it is rationally formulated by man himself. And just as Kant proposed that duties derive from human reason, so too, in other philosophies of the period, rights became detached from the amorphous promises of divine guarantee, and took on a secular form. The Doctrine of Natural Rights, though ultimately no more verifiable in its essentialism than its god-given counterpart, nevertheless rooted itself in human nature and served to mark the boundaries which differentiate individuals from one another. What is most clearly promoted and legitimised by the move to offer explanations and justification in human terms – rather than as a matter of faith – is the status of the individual as the autonomous agent of morality.

I am by no means suggesting that modernist ethics can be conceived as a seamless whole, and there are, of course, significant counter-discourses which do challenge choice and rationality as central to ethical enterprise. Schopenhauer, for example, rejects the notion of a free and controlling intellect which guides behaviour in accordance with rational and calculative principles in favour of a kind of compassion for the other;[1] but his voice, like that of Nietzsche in quite other ways, was a dissident one. Certainly neither plays any significant role in the discipline of bioethics. In general, the notion of a dispassionate individuality, with its component parts of subjectivity, autonomy and differentiation, is deeply characteristic of the modern conception of moral agency. Moreover, as will become apparent, outside the limited existentialist and phenomenological traditions, those attributes are conceived as highly abstract, not just detached from the sway of feeling and emotion, but from the body itself. Given the displacement of divine authority, the subject itself becomes transcendent, out of touch with the fabric of the body. And despite the recent and growing interest in phenomenology – which throws up its own problems – biomedical interest remains focused on the self-present, but essentially disembodied, individual who has been at the centre of both social and moral meaning in the dominant discourses of liberal humanism. In other words, there is a highly selective take-up of Kantian and post-Kantian philosophy which privileges a taken-for-granted founding ontology of personhood, with its implicit claim to universal validity, as the all but undisputed base of contemporary bioethics.

Against that static vision of self-evident, self-authorising and stable 'truths' the challenge offered by new Continental philosophies, and by feminist theory as it both precedes, reflects and develops poststructuralist insights, is faced by formidable 'methodological' problems. It is one thing to point to the actual existence of, or potential for, alternatives, but quite another to unravel partiality and historical specificity in order to contest the claim to universality of any particular system. More significantly, in so far as the challenge itself entails a rejection of the transcendent 'view from nowhere', appeal cannot be made to any external standard of veracity. But though the attempt to interrogate any explanatory system from within will always be an heroic task, we may take comfort in Foucault's observation in *The History of Sexuality*, volume 1, that there is never, even at a given time, one single, all-embracing discourse (1979: 100ff.). In outlining what he calls the 'rule of the tactical polyvalence of discourses', he speaks rather of dispersed discourses which run side by side, decentring the power of any one and offering a multiplicity of competing meanings and explanations. The very existence of these micro-centres of what he calls the power-knowledge nexus resists any attempt finally to impose unitary meaning, even as a limited historical construct. As he puts it: 'Relations of power-knowledge are not static forms of distribution, they are "matrices of transformation"' (Foucault 1979: 99).

It is difficult to determine just how far Foucault subscribed to the notion of a dominant discourse, and indeed he explicitly decried the efforts of commentators to impose any form of closure on his theoretical work (Foucault 1980: 38). He speaks sometimes as though there were no acknowledged centre of reference, at others as though there were at least an overriding locus of power; but it seems to me both counter-intuitive and unproductive for the project of feminism to imagine that all micro-centres are similarly effective. Indeed, the whole import of resistant discourses would be lost, and the idea of change would become meaningless, except as value-free flux. Nancy Fraser (1989), among others, has raised doubts about the efficacy of a Foucauldian framework for any radical challenge to orthodoxy, but I cannot share her pessimism. As Zillah Eisenstein puts it: 'Power need not be seen as a unified whole to be recognised as having concentrated sites that formulate hierarchical privilege' (1989: 16). Indeed, when Foucault speaks of the 'polymorphous techniques of power' (1979: 11), and details the way in which power infiltrates every consciousness – not through the exercise of a central force which brutally or repressively imposes a particular ideology, but by the operation of countless everyday and dispersed mechanisms of control – one must conclude that what is being put in place is precisely a dominant discourse. And as I have outlined in Chapter 1, the notion of surveillance, what Foucault calls 'the gaze',[2] is one principal mode of control. Whether its operation is through the institutional structure of hospitals, for example, or the confessional setting of the GP consultation, the gaze is characteristic of modern medical discourse. It may be either local or central, but what matters is the Foucauldian delineation of any discourse as a partial and specific construct. Moreover, what is expressed is never a given, never some inviolable ideal, but is always mediated, always filtered through not just existent epistemic values but also concrete social structures.

The twentieth-century contestation of the notion of self-evident, self-authorising and stable 'truths' is a common feature of a variety of philosophical critiques of modernity. In contrast to Foucauldian analytics, the more abstract poststructuralism of Derrida, and Lacanian psychoanalysis, for example, concern themselves little with material conditions but share a common belief in the construction of received meaning. The primary theme, which challenges liberal humanism in the most radical way, is that meaning itself is discursive. Thus, far from being related to any existent objective 'facts', it is produced only through and within the symbolic construct of language. Further, as I shall go on to outline, Derrida's deconstruction of the stability of meaning shows that it is not just that knowledge claims about the external world must be elusive, but that our selves too have no fixed referent. For Lacan, it is the entry into the Symbolic, the realm of language use, that makes individual differentiation possible: there is no prior subjectivity; it exists only as it is constructed by discourse (Lacan 1977a: 151–2). The problematisation of external reality and the linguistic construction of meaning are already features of Kantian and post-Kantian discourse, but those models remain nonetheless coherent, where the limits of the subject's world and the limits of language are coincident. What is new about recent Continental philosophy is that the subject is radically decentred, and rather than speaking, it is spoken by language. Accordingly, the humanist notion – particularly as it figures in bioethics – of the individual as a free-choosing, rational being in control of a system of meaning and value is fatally undermined. Not only authority and autonomy, but also the very subjectivity of the individual, the sense of the self as a self, is put into question. Similarly Althusser, adapting the Lacanian idea of misrecognition to a neo-Marxist framework, claimed that it is the elementary effect of ideology to make things seem obvious, to 'guarantee' for us that we are 'concrete, individual, distinguishable and (naturally) irreplaceable subjects'(1971: 161–2); whereas in reality we are simply interpellated as subjects by ideology itself, though ultimately situated within specific material conditions.

Now this sense of the inescapability of ideology, together with the perception that any critique must arise within the existing episteme and can have no external point of reference, is one of the defining points of poststructuralist thought. The claim is that there is no outside to discourse, no essence of human nature, no 'facts' to act on. The issue should not be construed as to whether or not a material world *really* exists, but that knowledge of it, and indeed of the human subject, can only ever be constructed through specific discursive practices. As I have already indicated in Chapter 1, what neither Foucault, nor other postmodernist theorists, seem to address, however – and this despite a clear fascination in some instances with the *féminin* – is what feminist philosophy has named as the hidden gender subtext.[3]

Undoubtedly, a continued gender indifference is a persistent feature of much poststructuralist thought, but that need not limit, I think, the feminist appropriation of its insights. Luce Irigaray, in particular, whose work I shall increasingly refer to, has built strongly and critically on the claims of Derrida and Lacan among others to offer a determinedly gender-reflexive critique of the foundational exclusions of Western thought. As her deconstructive trawl through some aspects of the history of philosophy makes clear (1985a, *Speculum of the Other Woman*), whether subjectivity is taken as given, or as constructed, the question remains, by implication, as to just who is entitled to function as a moral agent. The challenge to the standards of modernity undertaken by poststructuralism decisively undermines the certainty of such discourse, and those implications will be taken up later; but, as I have been arguing throughout, liberal humanist ethics is in its own terms deeply inadequate for, and often inimical to, women. Where, on the surface, gender is posed only as a matter of indifference or irrelevance, it is my contention, as Irigaray herself argues, that at a foundational level it is actively and necessarily suppressed. To reiterate, morality is fundamentally mediated by gender.

THE GENDER SUBTEXT

The explicit claim made for the mainstream systems of morality to which I have referred so far – and which are taken up in bioethics – is that their principles and resultant action guides have universal applicability in all relevantly similar circumstances. The conventional designation of 'man' as the agent of morality is supposedly a gender-neutral universal, but as many feminist theorists have now shown,[4] the suppression of the female pronoun is far from irrelevant or innocent. Instead, it is significant precisely because it reflects an entrenched and unacknowledged normative structure in which the gendered male is privileged in both the abstract and social context. The unmasking of that partiality of gender assignment marks the site of a major challenge to the unitary voice of Western philosophy. The intellectual tradition can claim neither universal applicability nor gender neutrality, but is throughout both structured by and the continuing support for a thoroughly phallocentric system of thought and action. I do not intend a sociological analysis of oppression in the present work, but suffice it to say that to obscure the relevance of gender and to position each of us as simply undifferentiated individuals serves to perpetuate the structures of women's subordination. As such, the dominant strands of modernist discourses effectively marginalise the interests of women and deny them a voice. And if, as Spivak puts it, 'the prohibited margin of a particular explanation specifies its particular politics' (1988: 106), then that is one reason why feminists should be suspicious of the theories of autonomy on which moral agency is seen to depend. As long as women have restricted access to both mental and physical freedom, and are denied the exercise of full rationality, then they must necessarily fall short of the male standard of moral agency. Even though, strictly speaking, such a standard represents an abstract ideal, it must be seriously discredited by its partiality in practice; and in any case the formulation that positions women as simply incapable of full rationality excludes them at a theoretical level too. In other words, whether or not gendered male and female interests and capacities are 'really' different at an essentialist level, it is the case that within the existing structures of society, those constructed values which masquerade as universal and timeless are just those which maintain male dominance. In other words, liberal humanism entails patriarchy.

Leaving aside the question of freedom, which for women is very generally compromised both with respect to the organisation of social institutions such as the family, employment, law and in terms of unconscious ideology, I shall concentrate my remarks here on rationality, the other cornerstone of moral agency. The claim that women are somehow deficient in reason – a claim that ultimately covers both degree and kind – dates back at least to the work of Aristotle. Given his ubiquitous influence on subsequent philosophy, it is no surprise to find an almost inevitable ambiguity among the major philosophers of the Western tradition as to whether women qualified for existential autonomy. Not only was the determinant criterion of rationality compromised in the case of women, but they were also in general more closely associated with the passions which the self-determining individual was supposed to transcend.

I am not claiming that this was true of all the discourses of the post-Enlightenment. Thus, Hume, for example, propounds an alternative view in which the passions are privileged above reason. Reason, wrote Hume, 'is, and ought only to be the slave of the passions, and can never pretend to any other office than to serve and obey them' (1962, *Treatise* 2, 3, 3: 127). In any case, a mono-lithic view of history is necessarily suspect, and Christine Battersby (1989) has argued persuasively that the late eighteenth century saw the valorisation of certain strong passions as a masculine char-acteristic. What is significant in her view is the way in which the usual markers of masculinity and femininity become differentially valued according to the male or female claim upon the corre-sponding characteristics. To be masculine was no longer necessarily bound up with rationality, but rather the claim to 'superiority' might rest in the male claim to such feminine qual-ities as passion. But it is only the association with the male that determines value, for if 'ordinary' women exhibit the passions it is a matter of their natural constitution rather than a moral attain-ment. In other words, the male appropriation of qualities hitherto regarded as the lot of women involves a certain transcendence, and consequent moral worth.[5] Indeed, in the period on which Battersby focuses, some passions were internally split (as it were) along gendered lines such that where imagination and sensitivity were appropriate to the superior male, the corresponding attrib-utes in women were named and derogated as fancy and oversensitivity. In short, far from resulting in a revaluation of women, the double gesture of male worth may have reinforced the devaluation of women.

For all the counter-examples, nonetheless, the enduring and dominant discourse, and certainly the one taken up in bioethics, has continued to privilege rationality. It is not necessarily that women have been deemed to be irrational, but that their ratio-nality has supposedly operated on a lower level to that of men. In being essentially unable to free themselves sufficiently from material concerns and emotions, women have failed to achieve either the ideal of detached, impartial rationality, or indeed the masculine and noble irrationality proposed by the counter-discourse of the Romantics. Men, on the other hand, were, in their own estimation, more able to rise above such mundane concerns, and thus were better suited for intellectual activity; able, in fact, to occupy, more or less exclusively, the place of the ideal standard. There is, in short, nothing gender-neutral about the Enlightenment 'Man of Reason'. In ethics then, the concentra-tion – newly conceived in the eighteenth century – on an atomistic morality, and on the notion of quasi-contractual rights and duties as they pertain to the self-regulating individual and buttress *his* morality, was largely inaccessible to women in both the abstract and material sense. It is not simply that the implicit and explicit denial of rationality to women may represent a simple category mistake, a failure of recognition concerning correct attribution; rather, as Genevieve Lloyd remarks: 'If women's minds are less rational than men's, it is because the limits of reason have been set in a way that excludes qualities that are then assigned to women' (1989: 124).[6] In the convention women lack not simply the *ability* to exercise full moral agency but, it is implied, the very *capacity* for it.

Now all this relies on an essentialist reading of human nature: one that not only posits immutable givens in terms of capacities, but one that is also fully committed to a conservative view of sexual difference. And moreover, it takes for granted the homogeneity of each sex. As a result women as a class are excluded a priori from full participation in the moral community – not just in response to the historical partiality undeniably in play – but theoretically, because a supposedly unbiased reading of essence reveals that it must be so. But who, we might reasonably ask, is giving the reading? To be valid, according to the conventions of post-Enlightenment thought, it should surely be some abstract mind able to transcend empirical interests; but as we already know it is merely man in his new-found, self-appointed authority extrapolating essence from his own experience. The man of reason, we must conclude, has feet of clay.

I have referred already to the predominant explanation offered for women's deficient moral nature: the historically persistent belief that the female sex is disqualified from full agency by its supposedly closer identification with Nature; that women, being somehow more fully embodied than men, are thus less capable of the rational, detached thought necessary for a mature personal morality. Whatever the putative cause, and whatever the focus, women are characterised as biologically non-responsible and suited only to be treated as objects, while men, by virtue of their superior rationality, may be self-determining subjects. Now clearly, such a crude division is further mediated by issues of race and class, for example, but a common justificatory feature of such discriminatory discourses is the link made between the body and moral inadequacy. The point is clearly illustrated in Sartre's existentialism where only the man, in the gendered sense, is granted the capacity to choose and act-for-himself, while the woman by reason of her biology is rooted metaphorically in immanence, is merely being-in-herself. Because of her problematic relationship to her body, she is never an independent subject as he may be, but is always the object of his gaze, the excluded Other.[7]

As an abstract concept morality is supposedly gender-neutral, but in practice its fullest expression within modernist paradigms is restricted to men, as they alone can satisfy its conditions. Biomedical ethics is no different from the general case, and given its grounding in empirical concerns, it may indeed reinforce the disjunction between women and moral personhood. As has been widely explored in the sociology of sickness, the tendency of medical literature and practice – particularly within state health-care systems – is to deny agency to all patients (Dundas-Todd 1989; M. Porter 1990). Such sociological accounts do not explicitly draw out the gender implications of those findings, but they do indirectly substantiate my own further contention that the relationship between practitioners and patients is constructed along putative gender lines. Clearly, not all doctors are men, nor all patients women, but the role of each is cast respectively as masculine and feminine. In so far as medical practice must deal with the breaching – even dissolution – of bodily boundaries, through infection, brokenness, death and so on, it is brought face to face with the anxiety occasioned by body fluids, which, as Liz Grosz says, 'affront a subject's aspiration toward autonomy and self-identity ... they betray a certain irreducible materiality; they assert the priority of the body over subjectivity; they demonstrate the limits of subjectivity in the body' (1994: 194). As I have already noted, such threatening fluidity is characteristically assigned to female bodies. The sick, then, must be differentiated from the well; they become the (feminised) other.

I am not suggesting that there is any conscious recognition of the negative coding of body fluids as incompatible with autonomous subjectivity. Indeed, biomedical justification for the denial of full moral agency to patients is more likely to refer to the possible pain and anxiety of illness as limiting factors on rationality, and I should not want to imply that those are insignificant. Nonetheless, my claim is that underlying such apparently reasonable considerations lies a culturally entrenched somatophobia which is most apparent in the response to permeable bodies. Now clearly, all patients may experience the real and ascribed loss of autonomy contingent on ill health, which for men may be compounded, and further constructed, by their en-genderment as female; but nonetheless, it is women alone who, in their inescapable embodiment, are held to be essentially deficient. The biological concerns at the heart of medicine ensure that, as patients, women are doubly disempowered both as 'sick' people whose autonomy is compromised contingently, and as the result of our immanent nature. The convention then is that men and women are deemed to be essentially different not just as a matter of sex, but in the attribution of moral characteristics.

The challenge to both the essentialism of human nature and the notion of a universal, unmediated and gender-neutral ideal can come from many perspectives, but the one demanding the most far-reaching rethink of ontology, epistemology and ethics, and to which I shall now turn in more detail, comes from post-structuralism. The intention of such a critique is to deconstruct the notion of stable centres of authority, be they the self-present male subject or the world of concrete facts, and to stress that everything we 'know', everything we rely on, is always already mediated in both perception and communication. The tool of analysis at the centre of the poststructuralist critique is language. I shall go on to show that Jacques Derrida's proposition that human experience is primarily an effect of language has a three-fold effect:

1 it mounts a significant challenge to the appeal to essential difference as an explanation of differential moral agency;
2 it exposes the hierarchical form of the linguistic difference which
  structures all our concepts and values;
3 it forces us to rethink, through the device of *différance*, the
  whole notion of moral discourse.

The feminist project of revalorising women has found much theo-retical support in the first two propositions; but, as I shall go on to show, the third is the source of very great difficulty. Once the very possibility of morality is put into question, as it seems to be, it is difficult to use poststructuralism or postmodernism in the pursuit of value.[8] Many feminist theorists have therefore rejected entirely or severely restricted their use of such analyses, but I shall hope to recuperate them for our own ends.

DIFFERENCE AND *DIFFÉRANCE*

The positioning of sexual difference at the heart of the feminist political and indeed ethical project represents an appropriation of the very concept which has traditionally justified the oppression and devaluation of women. Although not all feminist theorists would agree as to its efficacy as an analytic concept, I shall attempt eventually to answer the question 'What difference does difference make?', and to show that recognition of radical difference is a necessary component for any construction of moral agency which is to include women. As Gayatri Spivak puts it: 'It seems to me that the emancipatory project is more likely to succeed if one thinks of other people as different; ultimately, perhaps absolutely different' (1990: 136). The concept as I shall use it will be a transformed one. It is not the difference that structures post-Enlightenment thought, which some liberal feminists have attempted to reclaim essentially unchanged, nor is it the deconstructive move to *différance* which Derrida makes and which may finally entail gender indifference. Rather, my use of the term will lie in the shifting and strategic area between an acceptance of sexual difference as material and irreducible, but not (necessarily) foundational, and the notion of plural, fluid and local differences. It is a sense of difference rooted in the 'real' bodies of women but insistent on the multiplicity and incommensurability of those bodies and their experiences. Accordingly, I shall turn increasingly to Luce Irigaray, whose project to recuperate, or rather to bring into being, the embodied feminine as the radically 'other' stands as an intended corrective to the primarily linguistic strategies put into play by poststructuralism. The Derridean deconstruction of the Western logos has been nevertheless a decisive move for a postmodernist feminist reconstruction of difference, and though feminism has sometimes very different ends, the debt to poststructuralism is surely undeniable.

As the major proponent of poststructuralism and its deconstructive mode of operation, Derrida aims to strip language itself down to expose its fundamental mechanism which he calls *différance*. The genesis of his theory lies with the ideas first proposed by Saussure (1960, *Course in General Linguistics*), who claimed that language is simply an operation of difference, and that meaning is constructed in the differential relationship between signifiers rather than being a fixed property of the signified. It was not that Saussure actively denied the materiality of what he called the concept, but rather insisted that it had no intrinsic *meaning*. Indeed, the concept could not be isolated from the interplay between signified and signifier, which together form the sign. If representation is taken to precede meaning, then the construction of essence is simply an effect of language. In any case, the sign, *A*, alone could have no autonomous cognitive value unless defined by its relationship of difference to another sign, *not-A*. There could be, therefore, no understanding of 'male', for example, unless there was already an implicit distinction being made that a 'male' was not a 'female', and so on. In effect, all concepts are linked together in a hypothetically infinite chain of meaning rather than having any existence as discrete entities: 'language is a system of interdependent terms in which the value of each term results solely from the simultaneous presence of the others' (1960: 114). Nonetheless, despite their necessary inter-connectedness, each signifier is clear-cut and distinct, defined by difference and opposition. What Derrida, following Saussure, has added to this basic framework is encapsulated by the notion of *différance*.[9] It provides not just a refined concept of difference, but makes a yet more radical challenge to the transparency of meaning, a challenge that makes appeal to any form of essentialism untenable.

The meaning of *'différance'*, which is at the very heart of a shifting construction, is deliberately hard to pin down. It appears – and this is much clearer in the original French – that what Derrida intends is some intimation of the words for both difference and deferral. What he wants to suggest is that meaning is not simply a matter of difference, as Saussure had claimed, but that it is always deferred or detoured, always in some sense somewhere else. Where Saussure saw definition, Derrida's claim is that every signifier carries within it the trace of the other, the *not-A*, which must be suppressed if the particular signifier is to carry a delimited meaning. But though it may be marginalised, the other is never finally erased, and in Derridean theory closure is simply not possible. The most accessible explanation of this operation of *différance* is given by Derrida in *Positions*. Thus:

> what is called 'meaning' . . . is already, and thoroughly, consti-
> tuted by a tissue of differences, in the extent to which there is
> already a text, a network of textual referrals to other texts, a

textual transformation in which each allegedly 'simple term' is marked by the trace of another term, the presumed interiority of meaning is already worked upon by its own exteriority. . . . Only on this condition can it signify.

(1981b: 33).

In other words, in a network of indissolubly linked terms the other is always already the absent presence, so that complete totalisation and separation are both denied. In the sense that signifiers slide into one another and that meaning is being continually reconstructed, the appeal to an essentialist theory of meaning is redundant. The idea of definition in the sense of both epistemic content and fixed limits is destabilised, so that definition is denied even as it is established. In that sense, meaning is complicit with the very terms that it ostensibly suppresses. Spivak's 'Preface' to Derrida's *Of Grammatology* puts it as follows: '*Différance* invites us to undo the need for balanced equations, to see if each term in an opposition is not after all an accomplice of the other' (1976: lxviii). In the unstable economy of centre and margins which Derrida calls *différance*, meaning, then, is provisional, its boundaries fluid. And it is here that I want to bring together the two strands of my argument: just as the excessive and leaky female body threatens self-certainty, so too the leaky logos undermines ontological and epistemological closure.

The radical deconstruction of the familiar device of difference has several immediate implications for moral theory. In fundamentally undermining the certainty of the fixed dualities and essentialist differences by which we make sense of ourselves and the world, the poststructuralist move problematises the very basis on which so many of our judgments implicitly depend. If all categories are themselves unstable and the idea of rigid universalist divisions are untenable, then it is difficult to employ meaningfully universal categories of good and bad, right and wrong. The appropriate deconstructionist manoeuvre might be to insist that as difference *simpliciter* – that is, fixed and totalising binary opposition – is an untenable construct, it must be replaced by the plural notion of differences. And what this would mean in terms of morality is that any frame of reference should always be acknowledged as specific, contextual, situated and fluid. In short, what deconstruction unavoidably suggests is that there can be no absolute justification for any position. Far from regarding that

possibility as a dead end for its own project, postmodernist feminism sees in such scepticism the opportunity both of challenging
male authorised certainties and of avoiding an equally damaging
reliance on female alternatives. And it is the last point which most
clearly distinguishes the postmodern from the liberal feminist
project.

Before exploring more fully the implications of *différance* for
moral theory, however, I shall turn to another major plank of the
postmodernist feminist critique of liberal humanism; namely, the
exposure of the hierarchical structure of linguistic difference.
It has already been remarked that a characteristic feature of
the Western tradition is the assumption of dualistic values.
Throughout the intellectual tradition, classical as well as modern,
a system of binary opposites has functioned to support what at
first sight seems to be simply a clarity of boundaries and definitions. Now this thoroughgoing division of concepts and categories
along the lines of difference masks, in fact, as Derrida and others
have shown, a fundamental and often unacknowledged privileging
of one term of a binary opposition above the other. The latter
'marked' term is always in some sense subordinate or inferior, by
no means a simple counterpart in conceptual meaning. Moreover,
'in a classical philosophical opposition we are not dealing with
the peaceful co-existence of a *vis-à-vis*, but rather with a violent
hierarchy' (Derrida 1981b: 41). The classic split inaugurated by
Cartesian metaphysics is, of course, the dualism between mind
and body, which in turn grounds the opposition between ratio-
nalism and empiricism, reason and passion and so on, right down
to the traditional split, one might argue, between doctor and
patient. What emerges is a complex system of opposites set in a
hierarchical relationship to each other within each pair. It should
not be supposed that Descartes was the first to promulgate such
dualism, for it was, of course, already established as a mode of
thought in ancient Greek philosophy. The Pythagorean table, for
example, referred to by Aristotle (*Metaphysics* A5.986a. 23–26;
1961: 65) counterposes the 'Limit' and the 'Unlimited' in just such
a way, so that, as G.E.R. Lloyd claims, the primary term is privileged: 'it is clear from repeated statements in the *Metaphysics* that
[Aristotle] believed it to be true of contrary terms as a whole,
that one of each pair is a positive term, the other a [mere] priva-
tion' (1966: 65). Clearly, a great number of both philosophical and
everyday concepts fall into the same pattern. The oppositions,

pertinent to my own discussion, of science/nature, subject/object, health/disease and so on quickly spring to mind.

The initial step of deconstruction, as Spivak outlines it in the 'Preface' to *Of Grammatology*, is to locate the points at which discourses undo themselves (Derrida 1976: lxxvii), to uncover the operation of hierarchy, to show how the valuations of positive and negative – itself of course a fundamental binary opposition – attach themselves to the primary and marked word respectively. Now although a seemingly infinite number of concepts lend themselves to this type of positioning, what is apparent is that many pairs are simply subsets of generic terms, or have been ascribed to them. What evolves is a functional set of pairs which consistently privilege all concepts linked with one generic term over those linked with its pair. And clearly one of the most striking examples of such an extensive division – though gender is by no means the only axis of difference/*différance* – is that associated with the signifiers 'male' and 'female'.

It is not my intention to deny the common-sense assumption of a 'real' material difference between males and females at the basic level of biological sex, but to reiterate that nevertheless even that reductionist knowledge is discursively constructed. If we accept the important poststructuralist insight that nothing is given to us unmediated, then sexual difference at whatever level cannot concern us *simpliciter*. Judith Butler, for example, has argued in *Gender Trouble* (1990) that the dichotomy between sex and gender, whereby the latter is acknowledged as a linguistic and social construction but the former is taken as essential and fixed, must itself be deconstructed. What appear to be the givens of biology are simply not accessible except through representation in language, and once that has happened the operation of difference, in the sense of imposed differential values, is unavoidable. The two categories then, male and female, are always already loaded, and it is a matter of everyday experience and understanding to know that 'female' is consistently the marked term. The relationship between female/feminine and male/masculine is not perhaps always clear, and as Battersby (1989) has consistently argued, again citing Hume, characteristics such as sensibility and passivity which are seen predominantly as feminine attributes have on occasion been part of a male ideal. That is not to say, however, that the feminine *in women* is ever given the same positive account; and it would be a mistake, I think, to draw the implication that the distinction between a devalued female sex and variably valued femininity opens up new space for women. On the contrary, the use in French of a single word to denote both sex and gender – *féminin* translates as both 'female' and 'feminine' – should pose no problems for a deconstructionist. And what must be deconstructed is the positioning of one list of categories and concepts that attach themselves to male identity – typically active, strong, objective, independent – set against those associated with female identity – typically passive, weak, subjective and dependent.

However, it must be stressed again, it is not simply a matter of fixed stereotyping, attracting perhaps the accusation of category mistake, but a thoroughgoing programme of devaluation of the female set, no matter what attributes it displays. It may be of course that some paired terms assessed in isolation give a more positive weight to the 'feminine' characteristic – care for others, for example, as opposed to self-interest – but it must be remembered that the whole enterprise is contextual, and that what may seem an advantage on its own is a drawback in terms of the whole discourse. The woman who 'cares for others' is clearly not able to establish autonomy, in the conventional sense, as easily as the man who is self-interested. It would be entirely against the spirit of the deconstructive project to insist that each term, or indeed any term, displays closure of meaning or finds consistency of positionality. It is above all an exercise in specificity. What we can anticipate is that the general split which emerges at any given moment is likely to reflect a privileging of the male and of masculinity. And despite my reservations about dichotomising sex and gender, it is not necessary finally to identify the two. My claim is rather that the categories themselves and the boundaries between them are discursively constructed so that they may be either identified or radically disjunct. It is perfectly conceivable that one who is named as genetically male may not simply be regarded as feminine, but may become socially constructed as female, according to perceived bodily signs.[10] The phenomenon of transsexualism is one extreme physical manifestation of such a disjunction, but what is more relevant is the way in which, regardless of sex, groups deemed to be weak or inferior in some way – Jews under the Nazis, male homosexuals, blacks, and as I have already suggested patients – are often, at least partially, en-gendered as *féminin*.[11] Difference is reinforced and confirmed by the attribution of differential gender characteristics which in turn are used to justify differential treatment.

Now the concept of difference creates a tremendous dilemma for that liberal humanist agenda which is committed to the notion that all human beings, or at least all persons, are potentially entitled to respect as self-determining individuals. On that reading, once difference, and particularly a hierarchical difference, is acknowledged, it becomes problematic to apply universally such concepts as rights and duties, or equality. One stratagem which attempts to meet the challenge is simply to deny significant difference and apply a standard of sameness or identity across the board. Everyone is to be treated the same way because once the superficialities are bracketed out all human persons are the same. Thus blacks shall have the same rights to self-determination, the attribution of the same moral agency as whites, women as men, and more relevantly for my discussion patients as doctors.

The philosophical justification for such an approach, itself an essentially modern one, rests on two characteristic assumptions. First, it can call on Cartesian mind/body dualism which serves to rationalise the idea that while real differences may exist on a corporeal level – a biological male and female are manifestly not the same – the mind is of an altogether different order, and is non-sexed, for example. Indeed it was just this move which allowed Descartes himself to extend rationality to some privileged women, albeit at the expense of effacing the body. Once the mind is privileged as the conceptual frame around which social and moral principles are structured, and in so far as women are granted the capacity of making that split, then bodily non-identity becomes irrelevant. By a sleight of hand, a standard of difference (mind/body) is used to justify a denial of difference (male/female). Second, the ideal of sameness relies on some belief in a universal human nature, an homogenous essence which will become apparent once the irrelevant accretions of body have been transcended. But in poststructuralist thought this faith in essentialism is shown to be groundless.[12] In any case the multifarious variety of human beings display differences in ways which cannot be simply subsumed under a biological explanation, but which are the multiple constructs that grow out of lived experience. But to dismiss these as merely empirical contingencies would be to miss the point of the exercise, for what is being sought is some way

of establishing a standard of sameness to underpin non-differen-
tial treatment, not just as an ideal, but as appropriate to the
material conditions of the here and now.

Given the conceptual weakness of the appeal to sameness, the
alternative stratagem adopted by liberal humanism is to respond
by acknowledging that while groups *A* and *B* are both existentially and essentially different, they should nevertheless be treated
on an equal basis by extending to the less dominant groups those
rights and privileges which the dominant group holds. Those characteristics which might be taken as grounds for exclusion from
the moral community – gender, class, race and so on – are not
denied significance, but are reassessed as *morally* irrelevant.
Although there need be no pretence of shared attributes, or of
pure unmediated mind, the reliance on essentialism is no less
entrenched. The new paradigm is simply that groups are essentially different rather than essentially the same, but the overall
force of the argument is just as totalising as its alternative. The
assumption of group homogeneity effectively stifles any move
towards diversity as a standard, and ensures that the acknowl-
edgment of difference remains firmly rooted within the dualism
of either/or, and never both. And although certain moral and
social rights may cross boundaries, it is not the case that the
boundaries themselves are fluid.

Now this appeal to dualism (either *A* or *B*), with its intrinsic
exclusion of the middle, is, as the poststructuralist exposure of
binary hierarchy shows, by no means neutral and would be more
evocatively expressed by the formula of either *A* or *not-A*. What
is at issue here is that the referent standard, the norm against
which all else is judged, remains firmly fixed on the primary term,
and although that structuration is linguistic, it is fully imbricated
with the social relations of power. Effectively, the attitudes, values,
rights and so on of the dominant group are taken to be not the
partial construct which they really are, but a universal standard
applicable to all. Accordingly, despite the ostensibly good intentions of the liberal humanist approach, any group which is
recognised as different, as *B*, will always remain marginalised quite
simply because having a distinct identity is incompatible with fully
encompassing the principles peculiar to *A*. It is not possible to be
in the words of the catch-phrase 'different but equal' if the standard of equality is a construct of group *A*. There is always
implicitly, at least, one who is the point of reference and one who

is different, and that latter cannot in any real sense be equal. Indeed, whenever difference is theorised, other than according to a poststructuralist critique, it posits a unidirectional model. The unmarked or primary term – 'men', for example – is never defined as different; it just is the standard of the selfsame. In any situation, then, where what is expressed as different is a counter-identity, rather than a radically alternative identity, power is a property of the primary group.

The understandable desire of certain hitherto marginalised categories such as women, gays, disabled people and others to assert their difference *as groups*, to claim as it were their own separate identity, faces other risks too, for it seems to confirm that there is something essential about the divisions (Fuss 1989: 97). There could be then no effective appeal to socio-political conditions to explain inequalities, nor while the dominant group controls the discursive production of meaning and presents it as universal could that supposed uniqueness be revalued. And while the liberal approach would be nevertheless to grant normative rights on the basis of some relevantly similar qualifier, it is diffi-cult to see how this would be extended to full moral agency, the very basis of which is the capacity to make choices *for oneself*. The only alternative for any marginalised group, all those who are not A, is to attempt to become the same as A, to assume an identity with A and to forfeit their own specificity entirely. Either way, while the point of reference remains that of the dominant, the move of both difference and sameness collapses into the economy of the same. And the effect of such closure is, as Irigaray succinctly puts it, that '[l]icense to operate is only granted to the (so-called) play of those differences that are measured in terms of *sameness*' (1985a: 247).

One way of resolving the dilemma which satisfies the general aim of deconstruction is to attempt to move right away from conceptualising the issue in terms of a dualism. The first step, which has already been undertaken, is to expose that opposition not as a simple difference between two equal terms but as a hier-archy between centre and margin. The next stage – and it must be no more than provisional – that is suggested by Derrida and his followers is to reverse the equation so that the marginal term is privileged or is at very least revalued. For some marginalised groups, the call for a reversal of the established order of meaning translates into a radical political strategy which contrasts sharply with the reformist push for greater rights, endorsed by liberal humanism, but which relies on either assuming the mantle of sameness or appealing to tolerance for difference. Certainly many oppressed groups have seen their most effective course in attempting not only to claim their own identity against the centre, but in imposing different values. But to make such a move is either to fail to engage with the underlying non-discursive power which guarantees the master narrative, or, were such an enterprise possible, to settle for a no less partial alternative. To construct a counter-identity, and particularly one which has moved from resistance to discursive and material power, could only reiterate the economy of the same. Even though positioning might change, the operation of a single referent standard would be undisturbed and the structure of oppositional difference itself uncontested. Moreover, as Spivak has cautioned, 'reversals of positions legitimise each other' (1988: 249). A fully expressed 'methodology' of deconstruction is not content to stop there, however, nor to anticipate some kind of dialectic.

The third and crucial step, then – the one that is the most difficult to realise in practice – is that of the displacement of the very structuration of the binary model. What is called for is the 'irruptive emergence' of a new concept, not as the result of a dialectic resolution, but as one which cannot be understood in terms of the preceding binary (Derrida 1981b: 42). The apprehension that all 'stage two' discourses are still fundamentally reliant on a notion of difference rather than the more radical concept of *différance* should alert us to their theoretical instability and to their ultimate political futility/inadequacy. And moreover, it is in the rejection of that difference which is necessarily encaptured within the economy of the same that the postmodernist feminist epistemological and ethical project situates itself. Nonetheless – although the process of deconstruction has no completion – the move to abandon difference throws up what may be an even greater set of problems.

The operation of *différance*, it will be remembered, radically deconstructs all reliance on essentialism, both in terms of universal sameness or absolutely defined difference. It insists that no meaning is ever fixed but always deferred, always as it were sliding away in an infinite chain of signifiers. But it is not simply the loss of epistemic certainty that should concern us, for here feminism at least has a stake in undermining the master narratives of modernity. More importantly, when difference *simpliciter* is seen as just another construct, then personal identity, far from offering an authoritative base, is radically destabilised, or more accurately is exposed as always already unstable. As Spivak insists in her introduction to *Of Grammatology*: 'The text has no stable identity, no stable origin, no stable end' (Derrida 1976: xii). In being denied any reference to a fixed standard, subject positions (man/woman; I/you; all the terms of self/other) seem to deconstruct. If 'I' only exist by virtue of my difference from 'you', then 'you' are a necessary part of my constructed being, and 'I' can no longer claim the sovereign individuality at the heart of liberal humanism. What this appears to suggest is that self-responsibility must entail a necessary responsibility to the trace of the other in myself. Nonetheless, all those ethical codes associated with modernism proceed as though self-identity were distinct and secure, the certain foundation from which to enter into autonomous moral agency. By contrast, in the poststructuralist canon, 'pure' subjectivity, as centre and creator of its own enduring narrative, collapses, and all notion of a non-relational individual autonomy becomes meaningless.

Now such an analysis, straining as it does at the very notion of humanity's belief in the individual's own subjective authority, must seem to undercut the possibility of morality itself. In eliminating what Derrida dismissively calls 'the meta-physics of presence', we are denied not only divine, but also human authority: the exact thing which philosophically speaking has triumphantly replaced reliance on the transcendent. If there is no stable centre, then certainly moral enterprise must look for another basis. In staying with a close and detailed analysis of texts, Derrida has to some extent side-stepped the dilemma of an apparently infinite regress of meaning. His major concern is with the undecidable interplay of language, with uncovering grammatical and syntactical ploys which suppress the other, with celebrating the excess that escapes epistemic closure, and with throwing up provisional and multiple meanings. Occasionally a more sombre note creeps into his work as, for example, when he refers to the 'pathos of deconstruction', and though he has already occasionally directly addressed political issues in the past, it is his more recent work which shows a turn towards an explicit consideration of the implications of poststructuralism for ethics. In an interview with Jean-Luc Nancy, for example, Derrida spoke at some length of his hope for 'another type of responsibility' and explained the necessity of approaching it through deconstruction:

> if I speak so often of the incalculable and the undecidable it's not out of a simple predilection for play nor in order to neutralize decision: on the contrary, I believe there is no responsibility, no ethico-political decision, that must not pass through the proofs of the incalculable or the undecidable. Otherwise everything would be reducible to calculation, program, causality, and, at best, 'hypothetical imperative'.
>
> (1991b: 108)

As the interview makes clear, Derrida is gesturing towards a future task of ethical reconstruction that others might undertake. Nonetheless, the point I want to stress here is that it is the interrogative nature of the ongoing project of deconstruction itself that forms the basis for such an ethics.

Chapter 4

Feminist ethics

Poststructuralism, then, and its further development into a thoroughly postmodernist philosophy, represents a critique not just of the failures and inadequacies of liberal humanism but a radical deconstruction of the determining features of modernism: self-presence, reason, transparency of meaning – all those things in fact which constitute the Cartesian *cogito*. And once the much discussed 'crisis in modernity' is acknowledged, there is no escape either to the certainties of the pre-modern or Classical period. Although the critical focus has been on the post-Enlightenment period, the Western logos itself, with its roots in ancient Greek philosophy, is problematised as a whole, and particularly in its fundamental predication on full presence. Claims for the stability and taken-for-granted structure of truth are shown to be no longer reliable, and the authority of the transcendent speaking voice with its unmarked appeal to universality is stripped of its grounding. Accordingly, postmodernism rejects the teleological assumptions of what Lyotard (1984) calls the 'grand narratives of history', preferring instead discontinuous, contradictory and multiple discourses. Now it is precisely this emphasis on the notions of diversity, plurality, process and provisionality which has made the deconstructive move so seductive for feminist philosophy. If, as seems evident, the oppression of marginalised groups is coincident with some manoeuvre which allows the dominant group to claim its own discourse as universal and necessarily true, then the insights of poststructuralism in general lend credence to the belief that it need not be so. In opening up the cracks in any discourse, in exploring the leakiness of the logos, poststructuralism offers both an indication of how the master narratives might be challenged, and the assurance that alternatives are of equal, albeit problematised, validity.

What postmodernism has added to the primarily textual concerns of poststructuralism is a widening out of its focus to explore the implications of deconstruction and to trace its manifestations in a cultural context. If we take the notion of discourse in its Foucauldian sense to include not just the structures of language, but also the material practices which it produces and authorises, then there is no limit to the field of enquiry. The claim of postmodernism that distinguishes it in some degree from its more abstract Derridean base, is, if I understand it correctly, that the crisis in modernity is not simply an ideational one precipitated by the philosophical deconstruction of the central and foundational claims of the Western logos, but is an unavoidable concomitant of late-twentieth-century technology, including medical technology, and politics. It is not just that the organising certainties of discourse are shown to be linguistically unfounded, but that they have in fact begun to fragment in terms of lived experience.

It is not my purpose to explore 'cultural' postmodernity in any detail, but I do want to emphasise that the move away from a strictly textual analysis can serve the feminist purpose. In the first place, what becomes possible once again is to speak of power, not perhaps in the sense of monolithic structures, but as a field of forces held together in shifting but temporally analysable and contestable configurations. Second, if, as I have been arguing, the male order of thought relies – in part at least – on a denial of embodiment, then one way for feminism to proceed is by reclaiming the materiality of women's bodies. The place of postmodernism in this respect is deeply ambiguous for, though it would fragment bodies as easily as thought, it insists too on the significance of substantive practices. And if my critique of medical ethics is to attempt any different formulation, then it must take account of the re-visioning of bodies, indeed the production of new bodies, that informs the cutting edge of medical research and knowledge. Even without the insights derived from poststructuralism, traditional ethics – and the law which backs it – is seen to be inadequate to resolve the range of moral conflicts surrounding biogenetics and the new reproductive technologies in particular. And in so far as NRTs may be seen as emblematic of postmodernity, their inherent concentration on and problematisation of that which is supposedly most fundamental to the state of being female throws into relief many of the hopes as well as the potential dangers of adopting a feminist postmodernist critical perspective.

The ethical agenda is a difficult one to project within the context of postmodernism, but given the theoretical and practical failures of conventional systems, we may find there some responses to the problems so far uncovered. My critique has centred on the exclusion of women from full moral agency as it is understood in humanist terms and has traced the following.

First, the reliance on autonomy as a necessary and supposedly impartial condition for moral agency has been challenged on the structural level. Women are empirically restricted in the exercise of freedom, and even denied access to the conceptualisation of it, by the male dominance of the prevailing ideology.

That element has not been greatly developed, as it calls for a socio-political rather than a philosophical analysis of the power structures of phallocentric discourse; but the point is made that the present organisation of health-care systems, and more specifically of medicine, is deeply implicated in that structure. Hitherto many who are concerned to outline a framework for progressive health-care ethics see the dyadic interaction between individual doctor and patient as the proper and primary ground for the appropriate moral theory. Their assumption is that the wider socio-political context is implicitly determined by the micropractices of the individual medical encounter, and that the participants are potentially equally capable of moral agency as defined. In reality, however, such encounters are never unmediated but form part of the wider ongoing discourse which has already compromised the capacity for autonomy of one participant more than other. Most ethical models implicitly acknowledge that reality, in so far as they take it as the part of the practitioner to create (Seedhouse 1988) and/or respect autonomy (Beauchamp and Childress 1983). The professional is thus positioned as subject of his own discourse, set against the other as object of his concern. Given the structural reality it is doubtful whether any patient-other enjoys full subjectivity, and indeed I have suggested that all are en-gendered as female. Clearly, however, women are doubly disenabled by their status as both female and patients.

Second, the intellectual conventions of Western thought take for granted a mind/body split which effectively disembodies ethical deliberation. Given the prevailing beliefs about female nature, women are denied full rationality and are thereby disqualified from moral agency on the conceptual level. In inevitably falling short of the supposedly neutral standards of rationality, women are not deemed capable of proper moral thinking in the terms privileged by men. One exemplar of this move was the set of experiments conducted by Lawrence Kohlberg – and heavily critiqued by Carol Gilligan (1982) among others – which deliberately used male subjects only to measure moral maturity. Kohlberg assumed that women show different patterns of moral reasoning, and that their inclusion would 'bias' his findings, which nonetheless purported to chart the development of all moral agents. By the normative standards of the Kohlberg model, women – as Gilligan showed subsequently – failed to detach themselves from their emotions, failed to universalise their responses, failed to abstract the issues, and so on. In taking such criteria as affective detachment, universalisation and impersonal abstraction as the objective measures of rational moral thought, the Kohlberg model would seem to confirm that women lack moral maturity. A poststructuralist analysis, however, refutes any essentialist interpretation of such findings, and makes clear that moral concepts are temporal constructs, not givens.

Third, the fixity of difference, and its support for the hierarchical oppositions which persistently marginalise women and position them as the objects of discourse, has been both uncovered and opened up to deconstruction. The concept of *différance* exposes the denial of subject positions to women as a conceit masking the fundamental instability of all subject positions. And it shows the notion of autonomy to be an unobtainable ideal constructed on the mapping of untenable boundaries.

CHANGING THE CONTEXT

Now the attention given to the material and structural realities, to liberal humanist modes of conceptualisation, and to language itself has revealed the whole nexus of ideas around self-determination to be constructs determined by patriarchal interests. Always bearing in mind that *mutatis mutandis* the analysis outlined may have equally far-reaching implications for other marginalised groups, what is of concern here is that the perspective of women has found little or no place. Once, however, the prevailing standard of autonomous morality has been stripped of its universal validity and revealed as a partial and interested construct, it becomes possible to ask what alternatives might serve as well (or better). It is not, it should be clear, that the feminist project must necessarily seek to rely on an authentic woman's voice, but that constructs other than the dominant male one might prove more efficacious.

There are, of course, several possible ways of proceeding. An unreconstructed liberal feminism may agree that the notion of autonomy is limited, biased and even unstable, but nevertheless attempt to reclaim it by pluralising the conditions of its application. The emphasis of such an approach is on diversity and, although I take that to be an important corrective to the imposed unity of the male order, I do not see that it sufficiently contests the definitional ideal of autonomy. The claim that women are every bit as rational and independently minded as men reflects a whole history of fighting for equality that endlessly traps women within the economy of the same. A second, and far more fruitful, approach, and one which more fully takes on board the initial steps of deconstruction, nevertheless stops short at *différance*, preferring instead to problematise autonomy as an inappropriate basis for moral endeavour. But attractive though its rearrangement of ethical concepts may be, it must surely run into precisely the same kind of totalising assumptions that dog liberal humanism in general. Nonetheless, it represents what is perhaps the current feminist orthodoxy concerning the sphere of ethics, and as many of its proponents are deeply concerned with the area of health care, I shall give it some consideration. In any case – and the point needs stressing – it is not the task of a deconstructionist critique to *falsify* rival claims (Spivak 1990: 135). Indeed, I am already committed to the view that distinctions between correct and incorrect are purely conventional; that truth is simply one signifier privileged in a play of multiple alternative signifiers. What the feminist poststructuralist aims to do is to contest the adequacy of all dominant discourses by interrogating and problematising the grounds for their authority. It is not inconsistent, I think, to enter then into strategic negotiations with those aspects which best express the concerns of women. The argument that the concept of autonomy is delimited, biased and unstable is an important stepping-stone, but there is something to be taken too from the humanist feminist insight that autonomy is, in any case, an inappropriate basis for morality.

The charge is that the freedom to make and exercise one's own choices is conceived largely in terms of freedom from interference, which at worst can swiftly degenerate into a kind of moral isolationism. Accordingly, co-members of the moral community become 'others', competitors to the sovereign ego unless firmly assigned to object status. The individualism inherent in the autonomous ideal stresses detachment from others, the ability either to coldly calculate the odds unswayed by emotion or to pursue ends ultimately motivated by rational self-interest.[1] Though the assumption is that everyone is free to partake equally of the benefits of such a system, the strong and powerful inevitably end up highly advantaged, even against those others with a theoretical capacity for autonomy. The responsibility of living as part of society where all might flourish is subordinated to an ideal of self-determination that, at its most unpalatable, results in excessive libertarianism. In any such system, particularly where resources are scarce, as in the health service, the interests served are those of the powerful who are in a position to claim and exercise their rights against those of others. Clearly, even where the liberal humanist standard of equality functions, holding rights is not co-extensive with the freedom to exercise them.

When it comes to rationality and the consequent view of moral agency the intrinsic dangers are no less. What is to count as rational is logical, detached, impersonal, non-emotive thought that has transcended the exigencies of the empirical ground to offer abstract universal judgments. It is the kind of deductive thinking which, though it may start from a specific problem, moves on to extract only what are deemed to be significant features in terms of classifying the particular as an instance of the general. As an abstract cerebral exercise it offers principles and rules as a guide to action in all relevantly similar cases. But in formalising what may be a very complex situation – perhaps a woman faced with infertility is being asked to choose between using GIFT (gamete intrafallopian transfer) or entering on an IVF (*in vitro* fertilisation) programme – the demands of abstract rationality invariably weaken the claims of specificity. It may be that for the practitioner in such a case the only relevant criteria are those measuring the relative success or failure of each possibility in terms of producing a live birth. For the client, however, the issue may turn on such 'irrational' considerations as her own anxiety, the needs and demands of her family, her past experiences of clinical treatment and so on. Indeed, for the professional the question could be construed in the ideal as simply one of clinical judgment (though my contention is that it is never innocent but always mediated by considerations of phallocentric power), while for the client it is at least implicitly moral. There is no suggestion that most practitioners would see the issue in such strictly formal terms, but even where they are sensitive to the differential concerns of their patients, the convention demands that they find a *rational* ordering of priorities. At the very least, what fails to accord with rationality is trivialised.

It is quite clear that both the 'ideal' of rationality and the allied medical model of health privilege the unity and clarity of categories, and demand detached judgment. But in so far as each of those discourses relies on suppressing the diversity and connectedness of everyday experience, it will be inappropriate in certain contexts, notably in many and perhaps most medical encounters. The Cartesian notion of 'high' rationality is, in any case, susceptible to a deconstructionist approach. As Janna Thompson puts it:

> Being rational . . . is being able to choose and pursue ends, to carry out means, which are desirable and effective. [It] is thus a human ability which requires us to reflect on and use our imaginations, bodily skills, experiences, attachments. [It] is inseparably connected to an individual's way of seeing and doing things. People may share some standards and methods and goals, but what counts as a desirable end or an effective means cannot be entirely divorced from personal assessments and style.
>
> (1983: 14)

Nevertheless, anyone who fails to satisfy the given (male) standard of abstract rationality may be deemed incompetent to make self-determining decisions at all. Within the specific area of health care, it is clear that the reliance on rationality works against whole categories of people such as the mentally ill of both sexes, and against older men and women who, in the state system at least, constitute in fact the largest group of patients. The point yet again is that although gender inflects most experiences, it is rarely unmediated by other structural influences.

With just such considerations in mind many feminist philosophers have suggested that autonomy as a necessary condition of moral agency should be dethroned and replaced by a more contextual and inter-personal set of ideals which show greater correspondence to lived experience. Although the analytic underpinnings of such a shift vary greatly, there is a general consensus that it is, at least, strategically desirable.[2] Though the charge may be brought against some feminist theorists that that formulation amounts to no more than special pleading based on an essentialist belief that women are by their natures more rooted in the immediate and everyday, the more cogent point is that *all* social beings do damage to their moral aspirations by striving to achieve detachment. Nor, the argument continues, is it the case that women are intrinsically less capable of rationality, though it may be suppressed or denied; it is rather that the *standards* of rationality exclude and trivialise alternative ways of thinking that may be contextually more appropriate. Using the Kohlberg model referred to earlier, and taking issues such as abortion as a starting point, Carol Gilligan (1982) claimed that her tests showed only that women respond morally in quite different ways from men. Where Kohlberg had characterised this as impartial evidence of a lack of moral maturity, Gilligan showed that the women's emphasis on affect, context and intuition was simply ruled out of consideration a priori by reference to male-defined models of rationality.

The inferences that Gilligan has drawn from her own empirical study of moral deliberation have been widely influential and soundly criticised from both within and without the feminist academy. Her extrapolation of general principles from the particularity of women's response to an issue like abortion which is so intrinsically tied up with a specifically female ontology would seem to beg the question, but it challenges us nonetheless to ask which if any circumstances are unmediated by sexual difference. The difficulty for interpreters of Gilligan's critique is to avoid falling into an a priori trap of their own, implying that the differential moral goals exemplified by women are characteristic of biologically fixed and different ways of thinking. If, however, the implication of a different *nature* is firmly rejected, and it is acknowledged that thought patterns are socially specific constructs, then there is no reason why those responses should not be seen as more morally appropriate to the social context in which we habitually act. Such a shift does not commit us to claiming that the resultant 'superior' morality is necessarily characteristic of women, nor does it set it up as the only possible practice. The provisional claim is simply that women are, here and now, more likely to respond to moral issues in this way, and that that response may be the more efficacious in resolving dilemmas to the satisfaction of all concerned.

But non-contentious though this interpretation may seem, it does in fact set up two further problems. First, it is unclear whether the formulation is simply descriptive of an existent situation, or is intended to be normative. And second, if the latter were the case, then does it not appear to endorse a perpetuation of the conditions of women's oppression which – eschewing a reliance on essentialism – must evidently have produced the distinction between male- and female-associated moral thought? Similar criticisms can undoubtedly be levied at other proponents of a superior women's virtue, for in privileging the type of moral deliberation associated with the female voice *within* the Western logos, such theorists would seem to legitimate existing gender hierarchies. Despite the potential inclusion of males, Sara Ruddick's concept of maternal thinking (1990a) and Nel Noddings 'one-caring' model (1984), both of which have been enormously influential in promoting an ethics of care and responsibility, spring to mind as examples.

The general ethical model proposed here is not one that I can wholly or easily endorse, both for the problems outlined above and for the ease with which it can be appropriated by the uncritical essentialism discernible in some take-ups of maternal thinking, for example. Nonetheless, it is one with which the distinctively postmodernist feminist ethic that I shall go on to outline must surely negotiate. In taking on board some crucial insights of poststructuralism the model has abandoned claims to absolute and ahistorical validity, but far from being destabilised by the deconstructionist critique it finds strength in the notion of process. Yet the moral deliberation it brings to differing situations is no *ad hoc* response, but one committed to a moral sensitivity both to individuals and to community. Rather than an emphasis on the fixed framework of rights and duties, the system proposes a more fluid mutual responsibility and care as the distinguishing factors of human morality. That emphasis on mutuality is crucial if the feminist ethics outlined here is to mark any real advance on previous models. In the field of health care, in particular, at least some approaches already promote an ethic of caring, but usually in terms of the realisation of the professional duty of beneficence (Pellegrino and Thomasma 1988). For such medical ethicists and, indeed, some feminists, too often '"caring" is a shorthand way of talking about what carers feel and do rather than what care-receivers feel and do' (Graham 1993: 463). In such a formulation, the self/other status of the moral encounter is undisturbed. In contrast, the feminist claim is that the values to be enhanced are transactional and relational rather than autonomous; centred on mutual realisation rather than self-determination.[3] And I take that to mean not that self-determination should have no place, but that it should be one part of the moral process, not the end of it. The conventionally construed notion of a morality enacted by purely autonomous individuals following self-centred rules of conduct, or coldly calculating the consequences of their proposed actions, just is counter-intuitive to a workable social morality. It seems neither valuable nor even plausible to try to isolate an independent personal morality from the social context in which we function. The provisional goal here must be to acknowledge always the textuality of morality, and to encourage the self-determining individual to root herself in the moral community rather than abstract herself from it.

The aim of mutual realisation is to overcome the implicit and explicit objectification of others, and to stress that morality lies in the process of realisation, not as the discovery of one's own fixed nature, but in the sense of development as a part of becoming. As it further becomes clear in the feminist reformulation, moral agency is not simply a matter of choosing and following a particular course of action, but a more complex idea in which the existential being of all the participants is of equivalent importance. In the rejection of fixed standards of right and wrong, and in the acceptance of a more circumstantial approach to moral issues, the model lies closer to some forms of existentialism and to neo-Aristotelian virtue ethics – as exemplified in the philosophy of Iris Murdoch, perhaps – though those remain irrecoverably centred on the autonomous individual. The move away from autonomy as at present construed uncouples the new model from the rigid demands of rationality and allows for a more affective, consensual and non-logical way of thinking which better reflects virtues such as care and responsibility. The intention is not wholly to reject rationality, for it often has an important part to play in clarifying issues, but to challenge its privilege and re-position it as just one possible component of moral deliberation and agency.

In contrast to this fairly cautious and limited, though provisionally useful, rearrangement of the crucial concepts of liberal humanism, which leaves the parameters of ethics uncontested, I want to explore an altogether more disruptive approach more directly derived from new Continental philosophy. The position I am advocating is that of the feminist asset-stripper, taking from poststructuralism and postmodernism only those aspects which will serve our purpose and rejecting the remainder. That is not to say that I intend cynically to overlook the inconvenient consequences of a deconstructionist approach, but to suggest ways in which their development within what has hitherto been a largely male-dominated sphere of enquiry is neither necessary nor inevitable. Given that the methodology demands a recognition of the permeability of all boundaries, including those between author, text and reader, it would in any case be mistaken to see the theoretical constructions of Derrida, for example, as innocent. There is no impartial authorship and none claimed, just as there are no impartial readers. In a recent study, Tamsin Lorraine (1990) makes the point that the production of meaning is always a self-constitutive act mediated by what she calls gendered self-strategies. And although her major focus is on those philosophers – Nietzsche, Kierkegaard and Sartre – for whom the pre-given unified subjectivity of modernism is already under assault, she claims that each was nonetheless constrained, albeit implicitly, to maintain the masculine identity of the speaking 'I'. By extension, her thesis could apply equally to the work of more contemporary and self-reflexive writers, who despite their deconstruction of the *boundaries* between self and other continue to gender the other as female. Both Derrida and Lacan, for example, are notoriously attached to the notion of a symbolic femininity as that which, though not necessarily devalued, is excessive to and other than the male. If Lorraine is right that the theoretical content is delimited by gender considerations, then it must fall to women to redirect that content. The purpose cannot be to produce propositions of universal validity, but to represent different, though no less partial, perspectives.

DIVERSITY AND DIFFERENCES

The appropriation of postmodernist techniques of analysis by feminism is aimed, then, not at closure but at opening up discourse to a multiplicity of divergent voices. What must be resisted is any conviction that the recovered woman's voice is fundamentally stable or unitary, any more able to hold the centre than that of the displaced male. Among many others, Denise Riley's pertinent study *Am I That Name?* and Donna Haraway's ground-breaking 'Manifesto for cyborgs' both take issue with the all too easy assumption that there is a single identifiable category called 'woman', or even 'the female'; while Gayatri Spivak has consistently warned against an uncritical deployment of a post-structuralism which names 'woman' as *différance*. As the first English-speaking translator of Derrida, and subsequently as an authoritative commentator, Spivak has a high stake in the canon, but insists that our strategy must be specific: 'It is *in the interest of* diagnosing the ontological ruse, on the basis of which there is oppression of woman, that we have to bring our understanding of the relationship between the name "woman" and deconstruction into crisis' (1989a: 217). What is at stake for feminism is how to chart a course between the closure of 'woman' as a totalising truth, and the ungraspability of 'woman' as a paradigm sliding signifier. Despite, then, the necessity, as Spivak pragmatically acknowledges elsewhere (1990: 117), of having some provisional starting point, what is required of a self-critical feminism is that the construction 'women/are' should be a permanent point of contestation.

On a less theoretical level, feminists – like many other would-be revolutionary groups – have learned the hard way that though the putting aside of differences can be politically efficacious, such a move works best when the intended outcome is the formation of temporary, goal-orientated alliances based, as Donna Haraway puts it, on affinity and not on identity. The strategic need constantly to reform and dissolve such groupings without alien-ation, and without power becoming concentrated in the hands of the few, is one of the major tasks facing feminism. The move of either suppressing or excluding difference hitherto identified as the prerogative of men has often been explained, particularly by object relations theorists, in terms of differential male psychology, but it would seem that women too must guard against totalising discourses. Although my concentration throughout is on gender issues, it should not be supposed that the lived reality of either women or men can be adequately expressed if classified solely by sex. The postmodernist approach lends itself to the deconstruction of all the central polarities of liberal humanism, and if those other areas have been under-theorised, it is surely that the tools of analysis are largely in the hands of the white Western middle classes. A radical feminism, then, will not seek to replace a race or class analysis, for example, for those must remain important structural determinants of self identity, and, more to the point, of moral deliberation. And nor must it ignore the local and specific differences between women which in terms of everyday interests may be every bit as important. The danger is that of allowing the theory of *différance* to override the lived diversity, and disparity, of women's experience. Spivak takes the figure of the disenfranchised to point up the danger:

> she tells us if we *care* to hear (without identifying our onto/epistemological subjectivity with *her* anxiety for the subjectship of the axiological, the subjectship of ethics) that she is not the literal referent for our frenzied naming of woman in the scramble for legitimacy in the house of theory. She reminds us that the name of 'woman', however political, is, like any other name, a catachresis.
>
> (1989a: 218, original emphasis)

And the point is not to construct some hierarchy of oppression, but to recognise that our reasons for positioning ourselves as women at any given time are extremely complex.

Despite these reservations, however, I want to go on using, if not the problematic signifier 'woman', then at least the term 'women' in order to denote some concept of shared community. Indeed it is difficult to imagine constructing either a political or ethical agenda from an uncritical celebration of differences, and a move towards some partial connections must be a minimal requirement. Nonetheless, the search for common ground must take full account of both the markers of difference between discrete groups of women, and the diversity of individuals within those groups, neither of which could or should be erased in practice. Short of reiterating the phallocentric practice of silencing others, there can be no unitary voice which speaks alike for rich women, lesbians, disabled women, white women, mothers and so on, and the particular interests of each must be addressed. Further, each individual is marked in several different ways at once and her focus of identity and allegiance is fluid and shifting. The impulse to foreclose on categories of identification must be resisted, for, as June

Jordan warns, none provides an automatic concept of connection (1989: 144). There can be then no appeal to homogeneity; but n evertheless all women, I take it, suffer oppression on some level that arises from their difference to men. And although that oppression may be experienced in many disparate ways and is intrinsically crossed and interwoven with issues of ethnicity, class, sexuality and so on, it nevertheless entitles us to use gender as an analytic category. The problematic of a feminist ethics concerns the need to recognise and encompass differences – between women and men, between women and women – without falling into hierarchical or oppositional ways of thinking. Audre Lorde makes clear what is at issue when she writes: 'It is not our differences which separate women, but our reluctance to recognise those differences and to deal effectively with the distortions which have resulted from the ignoring and misnaming of those differences' (1984: 122). If, then, the real material differences between people are to be acknowledged, difference must be reconstructed as diverse, plural and in practical terms irreducible. It is not enough simply to avoid the false homogeneity of sameness, for simple difference (black/white, young/old, heterosexual/homosexual) is conceptually organised in equally homogenous and oppressive binary opposites. The notion of diversity, by contrast, embraces heterogeneity, sidesteps the devices of dualistic hierarchy, and allows differences and sameness to coexist and mingle. It takes on in short something of the indeterminacy of *différance* without losing touch with material circumstances.

Now, although a postmodernist feminism and a reconstructed liberal humanism both insist on the centrality of diversity in terms of a new ethics, their use of the concept is by no means the same. Where the former takes its cue from the discursive strategies of poststructuralism, the latter is more clearly concerned with differences in the wholly material sense. The simple listing of binary oppositions and their reformulation as unmarked diversities need involve little more than the political desire to undo the powerful hegemonic interests implicit in the socio-historical construction of modern ethical discourse. What is missing is any account of the instability inherent in the symbolic construction of terms. To take on board the full agenda of postmodernism involves, moreover, at least four major and interlinked difficulties arising from the deconstruction of binary opposites and the consequent problematisation of universalism which results from a pluralisation of perspectives. I have already touched on the first highly contentious issue which asks the paradoxical question of whether a feminist analysis which acknowledges multiple differences must abandon sexual difference as a category. Second, and this is a problem which may to some extent surface in a different shape in a reformed humanist approach, is the issue of moral relativism. Does not the loss of fixed truths and transcendence suggest that each account must be given the same weight? Certainly without some reliance on normative underpinnings, there appears to be no way in which to privilege women's perspectives over and above that of the dominant male discourse which has excluded them. Third, a whole set of troublesome issues concerning the deconstruction of subjectivity begins to emerge. If the notion of a self-present, self-authorising subject, the 'I' who speaks and acts, is put in doubt, then the issue of moral agency loses its transparency of meaning and the very focus of feminist enquiry dissolves. Finally, the project of making embodiment a determining feature of a feminist ethics is undermined both by the deconstruction of the discourse of biology and by the rejection of essentialism.

In short, the very language of morality as it is conventionally understood is problematised, and the way to effective alternatives seems blocked by the fragments. It is no surprise then to find that many feminist ethicists have concluded that the analytic strategy of postmodernism, while effecting a dazzling demolition of phallocentric moral systems, can only lead to a dead end for women. On the other hand, given the exclusivity of the terms of modernity, the turn to plural differences and diversity presents itself as an effective and theoretically defensible, though limited, expedient. As already outlined in its simplest form, the most common feature of such an approach is the willingness to abandon the notion of an autonomous self defined against a given other/object and to emphasise instead the multiplicity of selves in a network of mutually supportive relationships. In order to highlight what I take to be some of the shortcomings of what is essentially a feminist humanism, I want to look in some detail at how it emerges in Elisabeth Porter's recent book *Women and Moral Identity*, which represents one of relatively few sustained attempts to address the issue of a feminist ethics. Unlike many of her predecessors, Porter does at least gesture towards the postmodernist challenge, but rapidly rejects it as inimical to the project of women, thus forfeiting, in my view, the opportunity to unsettle the phallocentric agenda at its very core.

Porter's aim throughout her book is both to give a sustained critique of the existing parameters of ethical discourse and to attempt to reconceptualise the field in a way which will properly include women. She writes from an explicitly feminist perspective, but is clearly concerned that her conclusions should be of general relevance to the issue of moral identity – which she takes to be central – rather than simply particular to women. Accordingly she intends to set up 'a developmental concept of personhood that emphasises human mutuality' (Porter 1991: 5), and which will make a specifically feminist moral theory obsolete. Her method is to analyse how it is that women are denied equal moral status with men, and then to show how the concerns of women might be incorporated into a general model. Her emphasis throughout on the 'self-in-relations', rather than on the more familiar and static terminology of the 'relational self', is intended to underscore her conviction that morality is intrinsically tied up with issues of ontology. The 'being' she wants to establish cannot be separated from its moral context but is defined in and through it. Implicit in this construction is the view that male philosophy simply takes the self as given, and then asks what it is for that self to operate as a moral agent. Porter, on the other hand, takes an essentially dynamic view of moral identity, which, instead of positioning the self in opposition to the other, is interested in the dialectical relationship between self and others, and indeed between male and female in experiential terms. What she intends therefore is to delineate the middle ground as the site of synthesis and of a gender-inclusive morality.

In common with my own analysis, Porter addresses in turn the major bases of Western moral philosophy in order to expose the thoroughgoing dualism at the heart; and she recognises that that dualism results not simply in contrasts, but also in the gender-linked and oppositional polarities that support, nevertheless, an ethics which claims to be gender-neutral. This identification of masculine traits with moral personhood is by now well established in feminist critique, and Porter acknowledges her debt to Genevieve Lloyd's influential essay 'The man of reason'. What neither she nor Lloyd go on to do, however, is fundamentally to deconstruct the underlying dichotomies. Porter's aim, rather, is to *reconstruct* the polarities in such a way that, although the tension between contrasts is retained, the antagonism between contradictions is overcome. She sees strength in both sides of the equation, and while rightly critical of an ethics which bases itself on the male-associated attributes of rationality, individuality and autonomy, she is concerned that those should nonetheless form part of the moral identity she aims for. At the same time the hitherto marginalised female qualities of responsibility, caring and relational sensitivity are to be given equal status as the determinants of a moral identity that privileges neither supposedly male nor female attributes.

Having spoken of the need to achieve a balance between opposing elements, Porter goes on to explain at some length how her own conception of a new, improved moral identity differs from that outlined by Carol Gilligan (1982). It is not clear that the comparison is entirely fair, in that the latter's concern is not so much with the elements of internal identity as with the relationship between the male and female perspective, or rather the masculine and feminine as Gilligan herself names them. Porter's criticism is that Gilligan simply attempts to add together, in a 'best fit' scenario, the relevant features of both the male and female moral voice. But presumably Gilligan's concept could also be described as a balance, so clearly at this point Porter must have something else in mind with regard to her own solution. Her use of the phrases 'self-in-relations' and 'synthesis' serves to indicate where she believes her own theory is richer. The idea is that rather than just adding on moral characteristics to achieve some kind of balanced identity, the moral core will be achieved by a dialectical process which encompasses multiple and flexible determinants. Porter sees her path as synthesising 'individuality and sociality ... in that it takes into account the self, others, the context, and the contextual self' (1991: 169). Further, 'this allows a vast range of character traits, differentiated not by gender restrictions, but by a conscious affirmation of the sexual component of one's identity as a moral subject' (ibid.: 170).

This seems to me a far more satisfactory approach than a mere balancing act in that it speaks both to a transformation of the meaning of selfhood, autonomy and so on, and to a vision of sexual difference that does not already presuppose an oppositional framework. The difficulty lies of course, as Porter acknowledges, in imagining how 'all voices can develop without

the negative attributes with which they have been associated'
(Porter 1991: 170). The failure to address adequately this problem
– although Porter does offer a much rehearsed liberal vision of
more enlightened child care – underlies, I think, her own general
failure to interrogate fully the characteristic terms of moral
dualism. Her ideal of some kind of synthesis is predicated more
on wishful thinking than on critical insight and points to an over-
emphasised concern with material relations at the expense of
discourse analysis. Despite her consistent flagging of a constructivist view of ontological and epistemological signifiers, Porter
nevertheless seems to take certain meanings as given and stable.
Her method therefore is limited to an attempted remix of categories which will result, she hopes, in a new moral voice. But the
alternative which she does not explore is to deconstruct the terms
as they stand.

Now, if a poststructuralist understanding of language and
meaning is employed, then the implicit reference to some reality
prior to language must be abandoned in favour of the notion that
meaning is constructed discursively. It is not that the material
conditions in which the female voice is marginalised do not exist,
nor continue to express a powerful hegemonic interest, but that
they are underpinned and always already mediated by their
construction in representation. While Porter is concerned to
distance herself from any idea of natural conditions of
'masculinity' or 'femininity', her denial is based wholly on the
socio-historical rather than on the symbolic construction of terms.
One consequence of this is that she fails to uncover the ways in
which each term, far from being a discrete entity in opposition to
its binary pair, is dependent on its other, the term under erasure
(Derrida/Spivak 1976). In addressing the issue of modern ethical
discourse simply in terms of its powerful dualities, Porter seems
to subscribe to the notion that the *A* and *not-A* of difference
simpliciter really can exhibit both closure of meaning and clearly
defined boundaries between terms. What she fails to recognise is
that that foreclosure is enforced – but never secured – by the
violent exclusion of others at both a material and a discursive
level. In her refusal to engage with the economy of *différance* she
prevents herself from seeing how differentiation both in the sense
of epistemic content and fixed limits is destabilised, and consequently how any claim that the male voice might have to be the
stable and defined centre of moral identity is undermined.

Certainly the female voice, what is in each case the marked term of moral dualities, *is* effectively marginalised, but it can never be wholly excluded and as such always encroaches on and threatens to disrupt the centre. In this light a reading of the texts of ethics would begin to suggest ways in which the intellectual edifice erected by the 'Man of Reason' is no more than provisional. That tradition refers as it were to an 'as if' structure of reality; to a view constructed in accordance with male preoccupations and concerns, but one which can sustain no claim to differentiation, stability or universality.

Given that Porter would surely acknowledge all those latter things, albeit through a different analysis, one might reasonably ask why it is inadequate that she should work simply on the basis of an 'as if' reality. The answer, I think, lies in how far her material concerns inhibit her from a full apprehension of the nature of provisionality in the deconstructivist sense. It is not, I suspect, that she is unaware of the postmodernist agenda but that she feels its emphasis on the lack of stability and structure cannot serve as a basis on which to reconstruct a moral identity fully inclusive of women. It would not be too strongly put, I think, to suggest that this turning away typifies a certain kind of feminist panic in the face of postmodernism, a feeling that those who go all the way are being somehow irresponsible to the feminist project (Brown 1991). Donna Haraway, writing of her own project in science, but with equal aptness across disciplines, explains the difficulty thus:

> I think my problem, and 'our' problem, is how to have *simultaneously* an account of radical historical contingency for all knowledge claims and knowing subjects, a critical practice for recognizing our own 'semiotic technologies' for making meanings, *and* a no-nonsense commitment to faithful accounts of a 'real' world, one that can be partially shared and that is friendly to earthwide projects of finite freedom, adequate material abundance, modest meaning in suffering, and limited happiness.
>
> (1988: 579)

Calling this a 'necessary multiple desire', she goes on: 'All components of the desire are paradoxical and dangerous, and their combination is both contradictory and necessary' (ibid.). That desire seems to me to state a fundamental requirement for a feminist reconstruction of ethics too, but certainly Porter is not prepared to take any risks. Early in the book in her discussion of identity, multiplicity and diversity she sets out her own concern to 'explicate the contextual processes in practical morality and politics of the struggle of concrete, embodied selves' (Porter 1991: 16). That much is unexceptional, but where I cannot follow is in what she sees as the consequent need to dismiss the radical scepticism of postmodernism with regard to all forms of universalism. For Porter that scepticism entails not simply an open-ended proliferation of voices and perspectives, which she endorses, but also an insistence on 'fracture, discontinuity, partiality, dissonance, oppositional consciousness, destabilised thoughts and fragmented identities' (ibid.). Clearly, the listing of these latter conditions is designed to convey wholly negative connotations, and Porter cannot conceive, as she puts it, 'connectedness with others where there is an emphasis on the value of opposition' (ibid.). Further, the postmodern death of the subject appears fatally to undermine the centre of any proposed moral identity.

Aside from disputing whether postmodernism can be said to promote *oppositional* consciousness – and surely it cannot – the terms chosen are reductive, but not in themselves unwarranted. Without doubt, the issue which Porter briefly faces before retreating to the safety of narrative accounts, unified subjects, the value of experience and a controlled kind of multiplicity is one which poses enormous problems for any account of a personal morality. If subjectivity itself is constantly shifting, dispersed and fractured, how then can value be expressed in general, and how can women in particular ground a value system?

The first response to be drawn from poststructuralism, and one which I have already marked, is that although it is impossible to use the category 'women' in an uncritical way, this need not suggest that particularised, individual women do not have sufficient similarities to make their conjunctions significant and meaningful. What is important, and Porter would surely agree, is that these disparate moments should be recognised as sites of multiple differences as much as similarities. The sticking point, I think, would be the provisional nature of the conjunctions, for Porter seems to believe that to stress the radical provisionality of something is to say that nothing can be constructed around it. Where she sees the dilemma as one which cannot be resolved without resort to 'fictions', I would suggest that the project of deconstruction may be, and is, arrested at strategic moments which allow for a more grounded reading based in both the discovery and construction of resistances.[4] In half recognising the provisionality of the text, Porter wants to side-step its supposedly unmanageable consequences by reconceptualising the notion simply in the weak sense that things change, and change indeed within the 'real' material conditions of life. What seems to me more appropriate would be to embrace the idea she takes from Braidotti of 'constant dispersed quests for critical standpoints and points of resistance' (Braidotti 1991a: 15). As the subsequent reference to Foucault indicates, that endeavour may both liberate and enslave, but I cannot see why Porter, and many equally anxious theorists, should be willing conceptually to forgo the former in order to avoid promoting the latter. In any case, if women are already 'enslaved' within the grand narratives of patriarchy it is surely worth the risk of seeing how and where those narratives might fracture. The widening net of regulatory power which Foucault sees as the consequence of the proliferation of any discourse (1979, *History of Sexuality*, volume 1) – which I take it is the idea that Porter has in mind – is certainly a compelling and ominous image. Nonetheless, freedom surely lies in the ability to contest and change the discursive basis of authority as much as in challenging the material guarantors of power.

I am not suggesting that the poststructuralist agenda does not throw up enormous and complex dilemmas for any feminist enterprise. Clearly, the notion of a 'moral identity' stands right in the middle of the difficulty in terms both of selfhood and relativism. But although Porter seems to dismiss poststructuralism as an appropriate methodology, she does nevertheless construct a view which is not altogether incompatible with its demands. Her notion of self, for example, owes less to the individual self-given subjectivity of the Western logos than to a constantly shifting, though always distinct, personhood defined always as the self-in-relations. It is perhaps more ordered than the supposedly chaotic provisionality that postmodernism would suggest, but as a moment in process the difference may be more apparent than real. The issue of moral relativism is resolved, I think, in a similar way by focusing on the instability of the field rather than on the instability of the terms themselves. In her reconstruction of morality Porter is always anxious lest it should fail to indicate that one can hold a notion of the 'good' or 'flourishing' that at any given moment can be defended against alternatives. Her concern seems to be that within the context of multiple perspectives and diverse interests, it might not be deemed possible to distinguish morally between one position and the next. Having dismissed the contextual validity of universals, Porter feels constrained to stress the continuing relevance of traditional opposites such as content and form, concrete and abstract, and experience and concept, in what she sees as a necessarily 'reciprocal relationship between moral principles and contextual adaptability' (1991: 165). And even though, within her schema, each of us is embodied as a unique moral subject rather than identified with a transcendent universal subject, moral judgments carry no connotation of individualism but are 'predicated on some mutual appreciation about meanings' (1991: 149).

Now if, as I have said, the project of poststructuralism is not to falsify rival claims so much as to displace them, then Porter's move to reincorporate some existing criteria, while at the same time effectively redrawing the parameters of moral discourse, is entirely reasonable. My only argument with her here is that she has an almost knee-jerk reaction to the concept of relativism. As I shall go on to argue, that reaction is surely unwarranted – unless, that is, she has identified relativism only and wholly with subjectivism, which appears not to be the case. It seems to me that some degree of relativism is both inevitable and desirable – in fact of the major traditional systems, only deontology dismisses it entirely – and I cannot understand why Porter should insist that her own stress on sensitivity to context is something quite different. It is difficult to see why her recognition and defence of diversity as the proper ground for a morality, although materially contextual, should not be applicable discursively as well.

My argument is that while the relativism which appears as an unavoidable consequence of the postmodernist approach must be fully acknowledged in a feminist reconstruction of the ethical moment, there is no necessity to push its operation beyond certain limits. By that I mean that the implications of relativism can never be ignored, but that they should be explored for their usefulness to feminist theory and for the way in which their potential destructiveness of all value judgments may be avoided. Clearly this is a difficult demand for many theorists, and Porter is by no means unusual in her strong denial that her own thesis has any place for it. In noting this widespread tendency, or what she calls a 'quasi-ritual gesture', Lorraine Code remarks:

Even the most nuanced epistemic analyses, that expose the exclusionary, oppressive effects of 'pure', 'universal' knowledge, are at pains to show that contextualizing, or localizing, 'the epistemological project' does not, after all, consign them to the non-place of relativism.

(1992: 141)

She identifies the problem as lying with a caricature of relativism which sees it as a slippery slope that can lead only to the morally bankrupt position of anything goes, and which counterposes it not just to claims of universal validity but to rationality, objectivism and realism. Now, although I would want to look very critically at Code's apparently unproblematised use of those three latter categories (she is after all cautious towards postmodernism), I am in full agreement with her initial comments. She cites specifically the fear that a relativist position must be committed to a supreme tolerance, and that this would leave no way of countering a situation in which power became the only determinant of what was 'right'. Although she makes no textual reference here, she could well have in mind Sandra Harding's suspicion that relativism may be a manoeuvre of the last resort for a threatened hegemony. In a much quoted essay, Harding writes:

It is worth keeping in mind that the articulation of relativism as an intellectual position emerges historically only as an attempt to dissolve challenges to the legitimacy of purportedly universal beliefs and ways of life. . . . For subjugated groups, a relativist stance expresses a false consciousness. It accepts the dominant group's insistence that their right to hold distorted views (and, of course, to make policy for all of us on the basis of those views) is intellectually legitimate.

(1986: 657)

Now this is a curiously pessimistic way of assessing the efficacy for feminism of a relativist perspective. Though there may be some plausibility in the view that the powerful may contrive to escape responsibility for their own specific truth claims by pluralising the legitimacy of all truth claims, it nevertheless remains the case that the more distinctive move is one in which the opponents of pluralism are just those who seek to protect their own privileged value system against that of others. And as Code puts it: 'An accusation of relativism becomes a trump card to finesse –

and silence – any claim that subjectivities and contexts figure in the making, and *should* figure in the evaluation, of knowledge' (1992: 142). Perhaps there is some potential that the move, not to relativism *simpliciter*, but towards some extreme version of it, might debase moral enquiry, but there is no reason to suppose that feminism, which certainly has nothing to gain from it, would be unable to resist. There is on the other hand every reason to see in the relativist perspective – the claim, that is, both that meaning itself is relative rather than absolute, and that statements of value are partial rather than universal – the very tool which enables us to make epistemological and moral criticism of male-dominant systems. And nor should the acknowledgement of other subject positions and contexts pose any risk of subjectivism, for what Code characterises as the 'model of the monologic utterance, the isolated truth claim of an abstract individual with only his own resources to rely upon' (1992: 146), more properly devolves on the systems of the post-Enlightenment. The move toward pluralism is precisely one away from the moral atomism which might otherwise ground subjective relativism. What should not be forgotten here is that the ongoing feminist commitment is to a fully contextualised dialogue, and that must always ensure that multiple and partial perspectives are in continuous negotiation, not fixed and disconnected.

There are in any case two distinguishable issues to address with regard to relativism. The first, and less contentious one for feminism, of which I have spoken so far, concerns the applicability of moral judgments. The principle of universalisation which lies at the heart of dominant forms of Western ethics assumes not only the universality of moral sentiment, but demands that everyone in relevantly similar circumstances is morally obligated to perform or refrain from some action. What the whole debate around sameness and difference has done is to open up the field to diversity in a way which fundamentally problematises the application of the justificatory term 'relevantly similar', and to insist that no one can be subsumed under general terms except on an entirely provisional and local basis. The turn to contextuality – and that is really all that is meant by relativism here – as a necessary determinant of moral action gives force to a feminist resistance to the deployment of phallocentric moral power without, however, fundamentally questioning the validity of moral terms. In other words, a particular action may no longer be universally obligatory, but will remain 'right' in specific circumstances. Going further, however, to deconstruct the universal categories of right and wrong, good and bad, true and false, and so on means both that those terms can no longer be deployed across generalised bodies, and that the unified, closed nature of each term of a binary dichotomy must be put in doubt.[5] But it need not mean that the undecidability of the signifiers should prevent us from assertions of value at all. In so far as poststructuralist methods enable us not only to interrogate but also contest the theoretical ground of moral knowledge, and in consequence the practical validity of substantive moral judgments, it does so on the basis of epistemological and ontological plurality. The multiplication of the sites, sources and constructions of value does not, however, indicate an unrestrained relativism in which anything goes. The demand is not that we should refrain from saying that some things are indeed better than others, but that we should acknowledge always the impossibility of fixing that judgment in either time or space. And like all other binaries, the signifiers of good and the bad leak into each other, blurring distinctions and frustrating the impulse of a rule-bound mentality.

When Derrida spoke of the pathos of deconstruction he expressed not what has been seen as regret for an irreversible loss of value, but rather the insight that each and every statement of authority, including his own, is fundamentally insecure. In any case, the deconstruction of the value system of the dominant discourse might more appropriately be a matter of feminist celebration. What I am suggesting is that the values we already hold are just those which marginalise, which exclude, which silence others in a morality which is unable to acknowledge differences. The Western logos has not eliminated all types of relativism, but rather speaks from one form in order to exclude another. What is masked by the appeal to a 'neutral' objectivity is the highly perspectival base from which its own partial vision is employed, to very great effect, to efface the claims of its others. What the alternative of a feminist ethic must offer then is a re-vision of both the field of value and the conditions under which the operation of statements of value make sense. In short, a practical morality can only be appropriately put into play when relativism is already fully recognised both in the irreducibility of the ground of action, and in the fluidity of moral terms themselves. The instability of boundaries uncovered by poststructuralism does not inevitably lead to moral indifference, but demands from feminism an attitude of high responsibility towards the elaboration of differences and particularity. To deconstruct the view from nowhere is not to supersede it by the view from everywhere, emptied of all moral meaning, but to open up a series of self-reflexively situated perspectives in which the focus is on putting into play the most appropriate, though provisional, moral responses.

The whole point of appropriating postmodernist critical theories for a feminist ethics is to uncover the way in which values are constructed, not in order to deny the possibility of value, but in order to suggest new configurations that no longer function on the basis of exclusion. And moreover, despite the apparently wholesale debunking of universalism that postmodernism seems to imply, it is not strictly required by an underlying poststructuralist theory which explicitly rejects the binary structure of meaning that would position universalism as the either/or of relativism. Any turn to an exclusive form of the latter is no more plausible than that which it replaces, and feminism should not be uneasy that certain of its ethical claims speak to the universal. The very tension in the postmodernist requirement to respect differences reveals not a contradiction at the heart of a reconceived ethics, but a proper regard for displacement rather than reversal in the process of deconstructing liberal humanist morality.

None of these issues is fully developed in Porter's *Women and Moral Identity*, and I want now to go back to that book to bring into focus other features of what I take to be an ultimately problematic feminist humanism. To a postmodernist, Porter's uncritical focus on individual personhood and self-presence, and the concomitant reliance on the validity of experience, throw up further areas of disagreement. Nevertheless there are significant areas of overlap, for though I would choose to operate in an 'as if' reality only in full acknowledgement of the fundamental instability of the operative categories – 'self', 'other', 'experience', 'good' and so on – Porter moves in the same field of concern but wearing, it might seem, self-imposed blinkers. In effect, however, the substantive issues to be addressed are very much the same. What she is proposing overall is a feminist-inspired version of virtue ethics which attempts to avoid some of the more problematic associations of 'maternal thinking', with its uncritical interface with essentialism, while at the same time putting great store by caring and communication. The emphasis on the mutual responsibility of each member of the putative moral community towards others, alongside a proper responsibility to herself is, I would argue, a characteristically feminist extension of the conventional notion of responsibility from agent to field.

The willingness to acknowledge the particularity of moral circumstances is a general feature of virtue ethics; what is different here is the rejection of the idea that flourishing is somehow tied up with an essentialist or functionalist view of the 'good'. In relating human purpose to ideas of an open-ended *human* nature and potential, Porter means to escape the rigidity of a gendered view that inherently restricts women. And while the very concept of a 'human nature' may seem to edge towards predefined limitations, she is careful to set up a dynamic model which stresses 'the multicausality and reciprocity of factors' affecting it (Porter 1991: 85). Her intention is to move decisively from the notion of self-realisation as the expression of existing potential to the more radical view of self-realisation as a process of becoming, moment by moment. And yet there is an anomaly here in that she is not clear whether the process is one of discovery, of exploration, or of both. Though she quotes de Beauvoir – 'it is in her becoming that ... her possibilities should be defined' – with approval (1991: 86), her indication that rationality, articulation, deliberation and so on are human moral traits which women may fall short of, seems to rely on some notion of a pre-existing and ideal set of attributes. One response would be to say that human nature is both essential and constructed; and rather than see that as a contradiction, it is perhaps more in keeping with the feminist reconceptualisation of philosophical categories to allow both.

The question then remains of what is to constitute good human purpose (1991: 86), and as I have already indicated, Porter's model privileges caring and communication. The claim is that, for experiential rather than essentialist reasons, women are already highly skilled in this area; and in explanation Porter cites the socio-historical split between the public (male) sphere of abstract, instrumental, self-interested autonomous actions and the private (female) sphere of nurturance, mutuality and a connectedness to others. Without suggesting that she is wholly unaware of the overlap, or of the modern Western specificity of that dichotomy, it does seem that Porter overemphasises the gap between everyday male and female experience, which she sees as characterised by 'the rigid distinction between public and private' (1991: 134).

There are two points to make here. First, what she appears to disregard is the extent to which, to use Habermas' terminology, the lifeworld is already thoroughly infiltrated by the previously distinct values of the system world (Habermas 1984),[6] and, as Nancy Fraser (1989) would have it, vice versa. And second, although her distinction does have some cogency, its explanatory dominance leaves her with little else to say of the discursive construction of differential male and female bodies.

As an explanatory model of gendered morality therefore, the public/private split is of only partial use; but more to the point it could account for the putative feminist privileging of the attributes of caring and communication only if the domestic maternal sphere is held to be inherently morally preferable to the world of paid work and institutions. It is by now a feminist commonplace that men should be more involved in child care and other mutually responsive and supportive relationships, but the approbation given to such a move is not often extended to the case of women entering the system world. Porter is at best ambivalent, but often slips into a strongly negative view of their chosen human purpose. Despite her clear belief elsewhere that motherhood is not a necessary condition of nurturance, she dismisses childless career women thus: 'such a choice is not solely a feminist statement on women's right to reproductive choice, but is also an absorption of an instrumental, calculative mentality which insists so stringently on the rationalisation of time and energy that little place can be found for children' (1991: 100). This worrying reversion to maternal privilege effectively undermines Porter's theoretical preference for synthesis, for what one would have expected her to see as desirable is a situation in which both worlds were fully integrated, or where, at least, there were free, unconstrained passage between the two by both sexes. As it is, the implication is little different from Sara Ruddick's model of maternal thinking in which a new, essentially feminine, referent standard is set up and it is men who are to be drawn within an economy of the same, albeit one, in this case, based on women.

Even if I am mistaken here, it remains unclear whether Porter would wish that everyone, male and female, should display the same set of moral virtues. In other words, would each of us need to be not just capable, but desirous, of both a caring and an instrumental nature? Would we all exhibit 'rational, passionate selfhood' (1991: 116)? To say that, given the appropriate conditions, everyone has a potential for exercising some virtue such as care is properly against gender essentialism and reasonably non-contentious, but to assume that they would, or should, surely reinvokes a vision of sameness redolent of a totalising morality. It does appear that Porter has adopted some Archimedean point from which to decide which virtues the wholly enlightened human being should strive for. In this she owes something to Habermas' theory of communicative action in which our real interests are not those arising in response to a partial or biased understanding of the world – the maximising self-interest of 'rational economic man', for example – but those arising from an 'ideal speech situation', or as Porter puts it, 'a reliable inter-subjectivity of understanding' (1991: 131). One immediately wonders what an 'unreliable' understanding might be, and the difficulty here of course is that both constructs seem to assume a position outside discourse from which to deliver judgment. It is difficult to see how either interaction or self-reflection as mediated by both rationality and desire can escape partiality of vision. And in any case, though Porter does not remark it, Habermas entirely neglects to provide the gender analysis which would at least begin to explain in more than material terms some of the existing forms of false understanding. His implicit assumption, that we are all equally free to enter into uncoerced and uncon-strained communication in order to reach consensus on real interests, makes no acknowledgement of the differential access of women and men not just to concrete forms of power but also to language itself.

It is precisely for these reasons, among others, that Porter's consistent emphasis on occupying the middle ground, of refusing theoretically to privilege the female voice – though as already noted she is not always successful in her remit – begins to look a little inadequate in terms of effecting real material and discursive changes. In her forthright rejection of what she calls gynocentrism (1991: 34–46), and which she associates principally with a radical feminism based on 'reproductive consciousness' (O'Brien 1981), she critiques a political, often rhetorically expressed agenda as though it were intended as reasoned *philosophical* analysis. Often it is not, but represents just those strategic moments that arise once the normative power of existing polarities is temporally reversed by the deconstructionist project.

The majority of the texts cited here by Porter sketch out positions long since superseded in progressive radical feminist theory, and I suspect that Porter's real difficulty lies in the uncompromising rejection of masculinity as it stands. What is sought by more radical voices is not, in any case, either the replacement of masculine paradigms by feminine ones, nor yet a blending of the two. Rather, the ethical project is to bring into being a reconstituted feminine that displaces the gender binary altogether. Given, however, that the final stage towards displacement and dispersal is undeveloped, that the becoming of a new relationship of sexual difference is still on the horizons of aspiration (to use Irigaray's term), it is within poststructuralist methodology a valid, and even necessary, move to reverse the hierarchy of centre and margins. In being committed to a dialectic, Porter is unable to see this and is left with a somewhat abstract vision of how a feminist-inspired morality might be achieved. It is not that I believe that the discursive manoeuvres I favour would lead directly to the necessary material changes which Porter too would want. It is rather that the radical uncoupling of the distinctive polarities of male hegemony, rather than their reintegration in a balanced form, provides the moment, local and provisional though it may be, in which feminism can begin to construct its own agenda. And where that discourse concerns moral identity or agency in the substantive sense, it may indeed entail notions of human virtue. For an unrepentant postmodernist approach, however, that identity or agency has yet to be established, and a feminist ethic must first concern itself with the recovery of possibility from the fragments of deconstruction.

Chapter 5

Feminist theory and postmodernism

FRAGMENTING SUBJECTIVITY

Earlier in my analysis I identified the problematic for a post-modernist feminist ethics as encompassing issues of sexual difference and differences, universalism and relativism, embodiment, and subjectivity; and I have shown already how the difficulties surrounding some of these have led to a widespread reluctance to engage with postmodernism. A number of feminist theorists, notably Nancy Hartsock and Naomi Schor (1989), have gone so far as to suggest that the promotion of postmodernism by certain male writers represents in part a defensive response to the political and social advances made by women over the last few decades.[1] With this in mind I shall turn now to the issue of subjectivity, of which Nancy Hartsock, for example, has written:

> Why is it that just at the moment when so many of us who have been silenced begin to demand the right to name ourselves, to act as subjects rather than objects of history, that just then the concept of subjecthood becomes problematic? . . . I contend that these intellectual moves are no accident . . . . They represent the transcendental voice of the Enlightenment attempting to come to grips with the social and historical changes of the middle-to-late twentieth century.
>
> (1990: 163–4)

The idea here seems to be that where women have hitherto suffered by being excluded from full agency and hence from the exercise of power, a new-found female subjectivity has recently emerged which might break that exclusion and threaten the dominance of men. In response, the move to deconstruct subjectivity involves, then, not so much an anguished recognition of the implications of poststructuralism as a male determination to undermine the very basis on which the feminist agenda of revaluing women could be founded. Yet, as I see it, the apprehension that women are not best served by the fragmentation of modernist certainties, not least of the self-present, self-authorising subject, makes some sense only if no recuperation of the postmodern were possible.

In contrast, I have been arguing throughout that not only is such a recuperation possible, but that it is *only* the radical deconstruction of phallogocentric discursive categories which can lead to the empowerment of women in ways which cannot be collapsed back into the economy of the same. In any case I remain unconvinced that the liberal feminist[2] aim of wrenching the monopoly on subjectivity from the hands of men by simply exposing the partiality of the philosophical legitimations for their exclusionary moves makes any real difference to women. That limited agenda seems to entail at least three related concerns. First, if only the eligibility for subjectivity is pluralised, without a corresponding problematisation of its meaning, then a female occupation of subject positions leaves untouched those fundamental structures of power which work on the basis of opposition and exclusion, and which are underwritten by such binaries as self/other, subject/object. Second, it may leave unaddressed the differences between women. That danger is succinctly summarised by Judith Butler when she writes: 'The premature insistence on a stable subject of feminism, understood as a seamless category of women, inevitably generates multiple refusals to accept the category' (1990: 4). Finally, the anxiety occasioned by deconstruction seems misplaced, for in so far as women have not yet in fact come to claim full subjectivity and agency, the crisis in modernity, centred on the so-called death of the author, is fundamentally a male crisis. And moreover, as black and Third World feminists are making plain, that crisis concerns white subjectivity.[3] At this point in time it is difficult to see quite what it is that women have to lose, for although those of us in the West may enjoy some social and political gains of limited worth, those gains are merely granted within a system that epitomises and perpetuates phallocentric power.

The discursive approach that I favour makes no claims to a social efficacy which could directly put in motion institutional change, but it does set up a space from within which women can both resist and deconstruct dominant subject positions. The aim is not to demonstrate how to behave as a moral agent, but to uncover the conditions in which moral agency is possible, if at all. What is at stake is not that women are discriminated against either here or elsewhere, but that within the patriarchy, as it coexists with liberal humanism, it makes no real sense on the discursive level to speak of women's moral agency at all. The task then, of addressing the issue of a specifically feminist ethics – such as might be formulated for health care – must encompass always much broader questions of epistemology and ontology; that is, questions regarding subjectivity. The issues are inextricably bound together, for to be a subject is to be, potentially, a moral agent, and that is one who is capable of making choices and acting on them within a given system of values. To be a subject is to be able to construct and define moral values. And to be a subject is to be valorised as a moral agent. In other words, the significant moment in the construction and operation of moral discourse, indeed any discourse, is the positioning of its subject.

To recapitulate briefly the relevant features of the dominant post-Enlightenment theories of ethics: the humanist moral subject, theorised as an ideal, abstract, quasi-transcendent, non-gendered 'person', is in practice invariably gendered as male. And for all the more or less careful emphasis on defining a category of neutral persons whose linking feature is an attribute of mind – non-sexed, of course – as opposed to any characteristic (inevitably sexed) of body, the parameters used are just those which intrinsically exclude women. To extend to subjectivity itself Kant's notion of the necessary features of personhood – as opposed to mere humanity – points to autonomy and rationality as the limiting factors; and both those features, though posed as impartial objective standards, are markers of a masculine referent standard. And within the systems of hierarchically arranged dualities which characterise Western thought, women are in effect disqualified from full subjectivity by the very condition of their embodied femininity and thereby excluded from moral agency. In short, the enterprise of establishing subjectivity implicitly relies not simply on the attribution of certain standards to men alone but also on a necessary exclusion of the subject's putative others, those who are objectified, paradigmatically those women. The conventional subject of biomedical ethics turns on just such a distinction. What the dominant modern Western notion of subjectivity entails – and it matters little whether the discourse is that of deontology, utilitarianism, neo-Aristotelianism or some other – is the concept of a free and rational sovereign individual, aware of himself as a self, and claiming some kind of authority, whether sanctioned transcendentally or materially, over those 'others' who are disqualified. In the thoroughgoing pattern of dualistic polarities which operate as power differentials, and in which the foundational distinction between male and female authorises an infinite set of binary differences based on supposedly natural masculine and feminine qualities, women are perceived as falling outside the closure of moral agency. They can at best be accorded rights, interests and even consideration, but in the final analysis they are not actors but are merely acted upon. This is not to say, of course, that women do not participate in the minutiae of moral life nor make their own discrete decisions as agents, but that so long as those choices are made within a liberal humanist framework which, in effect, entails denial of female subjectivity, then they cannot properly be said to be moral acts within the given terms of that system. Women do not set their own standards of reference, but act and react according to the masculine ideal.

The agenda for feminist ethics, then, revolves round issues of sameness and difference. Indeed, to be a modern subject, to be a moral agent in one's own right, is a matter of taking on the ontological status of a man. And to be the same as a man is to be no less than a man. To be different is to fall short; to be not so much woman as not-man; to be the other whose very (non)presence confirms, as Luce Irigaray argues (1985a: *passim*), the unity and self-identity of the masculine subject. Men, of course, are never spoken of as different, or even the same; they simply are the standard which is both ideal and normative. Effectively, to be valorised is to be male. Both sameness and difference effectively silence women in their sexual specificity and render a female subjectivity impossible.

Historically the liberal feminist response to the inevitable, and indeed necessary, failure of women in general to make the grade is to claim that if only they were better supported in terms of education, legal rights, material stability and so on, then they would indeed be equal to men. What constitutes the problem as they see it is that women are debarred, not because of any intrinsic failing, but because men have occupied the place of subjectivity and unfairly, partially, used their power to ensure that women will fail to satisfy the entrance requirements. As, however, such an account fails to thematise the whole epistemological structure of difference, it leaves open the possibility for men to go on claiming that women's exclusion from full personhood hangs on their *essential* inability to exercise independence and rationality. Thus, either a woman's best hope lies in her identification with the standard of sameness, or she must accept that she is essentially, irretrievably, different, and in opposition to the masculine. What is missing from such an analysis seems to be any awareness of how it is not just that dominant males occupy the place of subjectivity, as though it were neutral and open, but also that they construct its determinants in their own image. They claim subjectivity as a personal property. As the founding moment of liberal humanist discourse, the *cogito* resonates with attributes always already coextensive with the masculine ego: self-presence, unity, transcendence, disembodied rationality and autonomy. And once the standard of subjectivity is privileged in this way, then women will always be conceived as the negative pole. Neither personhood nor the notion of the transcendental subject is fully open to women.

Against that project of modernity centred on the unified masculine subject, the sustained and damaging critique put into play by the insights of various strands of poststructuralism has fundamentally contested the very ontological status of conventional notions of subjectivity. And it is here that we may find our best opportunity as women of breaking free of the male monopoly on meaning, and of finding validation in/for the discourse of the other. What is at stake, though not surprisingly under-theorised by the founder-masters of poststructuralism,[4] is who is at the centre of language – the medium of discursive construction which has appeared to guarantee patriarchal power.

The postmodernist feminist contention that subjectivity is always already gendered (Butler 1991: 24; Flax 1992: 455) nonetheless builds on such male-authored and apparently gender-indifferent accounts. In particular, Foucault's notion of power/knowledge as that which precedes and constitutes subjectivity provides fertile ground for a specifically feminist problematisation of the subject. Unlike Derrida, whose concentration is on the linguistic structures which buttress subjectivity, Foucault traces its discursive construction both through that which is spoken and through material practices:

we should try to discover how it is that subjects are gradually, progressively, really and materially constituted through a multiplicity of organisms, forces, energies, materials, desires, thoughts etc. We should try to grasp subjection in its material instance as a constitution of subjects.

(1980: 97)

In the early and middle works at least, to become a subject, then, is to be subjected to some force or power which constructs even as it seeks to control. In the same way that the various technologies of domination are not directed at pre-existing bodies (as I have outlined in Chapter 1), so too there are no pre-existing subjects. As Foucault puts it: 'The body is the inscribed surface of events (traced by language and dissolved by ideas), the locus of a dissociated self (adopting the illusion of a substantial unity)' (1977b: 148). Subjectivity, in other words, is not the manifest property of an interior self but merely a more or less unstable effect of power. And that for feminism must indicate the liberatory potential to refuse the assignment of our identities by the dominant discourse.

The great difficulty for any political or ethical agenda with that formulation is that it seems to speak only to an inescapable lack of agency on the part of any individual. Certainly transformation is a consistent feature of the tenure of subjectivity, but it is not clear how strategies of resistance can be directed in any particular way. That lack of prior determination should not, however, vitiate the efficacy of resistance to technologies of power, but we must be prepared to embrace some risk in that the outcome is never certain. Towards the end of his career Foucault suggested ways in which the techniques of domination that instantiate and regulate subjects might be offset by what he called 'the practices of the self' (1985b; 1986). Without repudiating the process of inscription on the open surface of the body, Foucault gave new emphasis in his study of certain aspects of antiquity to the possibilities of self-determination through a reflexive stylisation which could counter external power, and which finds its ethical moment in self-restraint. I find myself unconvinced that this new turn to the place of self-discipline is anything more than a restatement of the way in which the disciplines of the body are internalised, and as such represent not resistance, but that which must be resisted. Moreover, to make, as Foucault does, the care of the self the new linchpin of ethics is to seem to speak to a nostalgia for the quasi-autonomous sovereign subject, the very entity which had earlier been deconstructed. Foucault himself explicitly denies such a move (1988: 50), but in doing so he must surely abandon the notion of self-determination. In any case, the original formulation of the subject is fully consonant with a self-constituting, albeit indeterminate, resistance to power: 'once power produces this effect, there inevitably emerge the responding claims and affirmations, those of one's body against power' (Foucault 1980: 56). It is not that the subject is ever emancipated, but that the liberties of the individual are both transitory and discontinuous, and there to be grasped in the resistance that power itself throws up. Nor can there be any *telos* of completed personhood, for the process is symbiotic and self-perpetuating, but never fixed nor unidirectional.

Moreover, as I understand it, there is in any case no real distinction to be made between subject and object, for both the one who acts and the one who is acted upon are constituted by the same range of disciplinary forces directed at the individual body. If, as I have claimed earlier, health-care professionals are the agents of a project of normalisation, that is not to say that they are not also normalised. The implication must be that relations of power, at the micro-level at least, are conventional rather than determined, and as such are open to contestation. In any hierarchical relationship then – and this would clearly include that usually understood to exist between health practitioner and patient – the overt deployment of power/knowledge is no guarantee of the security of the place of the subject. It is something of a commonplace to point to the social construction of health and disease using a Foucauldian analysis (Armstrong 1983; Turner 1987), but that usually rests on the pre-critical assumption of existent subjects on whom to mark those categories. Nicholas Fox is rare among the theorists of health care in making the further step when he comments that what is usually achieved in curing is 'a fabricated, contingent, partial, local, social, figuration of power/knowledge, constitutive of a particular subjectivity of health and illness' (1993: 58). And I would want to extend that deconstructive move to challenge not simply the fixity of the relationship between health and disease, but between the subject and object of those discourses however they are manifested.

As I have already outlined, the Derridean approach entails a close interrogation both of difference and of those exclusionary procedures which underwrite the enduring stability of all categories. In the deconstruction of the structure of difference, and the move into *différance*, what has disappeared is any fixed point of reference which represents or corresponds to some given transcendent reality. Not only does representation precede meaning, but the primary term is both literally meaningless without the margins of its own discourse, and unable to erase the trace of its others. What that means in terms of the subject is that the self does not precede its differentiation from the other – the multiple others homogenised here into a single category – but is founded in the very project of setting boundaries. It is not that language is ever made entirely unusable by the slide of signifiers; clearly we do go on using it to communicate with one another, most notably by the extensive use of the referent 'I'. But what can no longer be justified *in theory* is the reliance on it as the guarantor of the presence and unity of the subject. The 'I', the supposedly sovereign, timeless and self-identical individual of liberal humanist discourse is exposed as (1) just another signifier reliant for even provisional definition on its other, the 'you', and (2) as radically incorporating the trace of that other which will always frustrate the claim to purity and autonomy of the primary term.

Given that my interest lies in the constitution of subjectivity through linguistic and social practices rather than in its interior emergence, I do not intend to offer any close reading of psychoanalysis. Nonetheless, it is worth noting that in Lacanian theory, in common with poststructuralism, the subject is not given but discursively founded on exclusion, and in this case on misrecognition (Lacan 1977b, 'The mirror stage'). The subject for Lacan is never identical to itself, but is always split. Moreover, in taking up a place within the Symbolic, the realm of culture and language, the speaking subject is not the origin of speech but functions only as the privileged construct of socio-linguistic forces.[5] As such it operates within the Symbolic only at the cost of the psychic insecurity of a fundamental repression which may always erupt into consciousness. Given the emphasis put on desire in Lacanian psychoanalysis, it might seem that what is added to the perspectives already discussed is a sense of the subject as constituted by something more than (con)textual strategies. The libidinal forces which manifest as desire do not imply, however, a motivating positivity arising from the body itself, but are linguistically constructed, and, as I have remarked before, that desire is predicated on lack. It is difficult then to conceptualise it as resistant or productive, and many feminist philosophers, notably Rosi Braidotti (1991a), have preferred the Deleuzean notion of bodies as active 'desiring machines' where the only lack is that of a fixed subject. Nonetheless, though the Lacanian explanation of subjectivity, especially as it is – and must be – gendered by the differential male/female relation to the phallus, offers limited scope for resignification, it does reiterate the challenge to the foundational 'I'.

It is on the basis of just such points derived from both Derrida and Lacan that Luce Irigaray takes up the question of the subject in a deconstructive *tour de force* directed at the whole structuration of Western philosophy. What she intends to show is that the very concept of an autonomous subject central to that discourse is a masculine prerogative from which the *féminin* is necessarily absent. The detached, abstract 'I', which Irigaray identifies as not merely the Cartesian subject but as a transhistorical entity (1985a, 'Any theory of the subject'), is constituted on the denial of the original dependency on and attachment to the maternal body. That denial is played out in the Symbolic as a generalised effacement of the *féminin*, or as the positioning of women as the reflective other of male subjectivity. What Irigaray claims is not that dominant men construct hierarchies which suppress female subjectivity, but that the structure of the subject itself relies on a gendered exclusion. It is not possible then to reclaim a *female* subject as such from within the system.

Now all these discourses clearly have immense implications, not just for the masculine subject whose claim to self identity has traditionally been confirmed by liberal humanism, but who now is shown to exist only by virtue of his excluded others, but for the whole humanist project of subjectivity. If the subject is no longer unified, stable and transcendent, then clearly the central figure of the dominant ethical discourse is in disarray. The question we must now ask becomes: how can this be good news for women? What are we to make of the feminist project of valorising women, of claiming subjectivity for ourselves, in the context of the radical deconstruction of the subject *per se*? Is there in fact any way in which we can reconstruct not subjectivity as it has been previously understood, and which is now in crisis, but a new feminist-friendly form which will answer to the specificity of women, and, by extension, to that of men too?

What I am suggesting is that a distinction should be made between subjectivity as a kind of fixed personal attribute held and carried by an individual subject, and subject positions as the diverse, multiple and local possibilities in and out of which an individual is both constructed and may construct her life. While the move to deconstruct the subject as a founding concept of Western ontology, epistemology and ethics may generate anxiety among some feminists and seem to undermine the very basis of their endeavour, it is a move, nevertheless, which is profoundly misunderstood. And indeed, even a committed postmodernist such as Susan Hekman, who wholly approves the Derridean project, seems to misconstrue its purpose when she chastises those who would seek to reclaim elements of the Cartesian subject in the interests of retaining agency (Hekman 1990: 81). I would agree with Hekman that anxious feminists have failed to displace the apparent dichotomy between the active, constituting subject and the passive constituted self, but she too seems consistently guilty of dichotomous thinking in her insistence on the either/or of modernism and postmodernism. In any case, the whole point of the poststructuralist approach, as both Derrida, particularly in the 'Afterword' to *Limited Inc* (1988) and in 'Eating well' (1991b), and Spivak (1990: 46, 135) have consistently underlined, is not to destroy or falsify the cherished concepts of modernism so much as to expose the slippage in their supposedly foundational status.

Moreover, as Judith Butler points out '[t]o deconstruct the subject of feminism is not . . . to censure its usage' (1992, 'Contingent foundations': 16). In other words, what is at stake is the claim that the subject is pre-given, either in the sense of preceding representation or of preceding the operation of power. Butler takes the view that it is the very grammatical structure of language, that presupposes an existing subject of discourse, which gives rise to such persistent claims that it could not be otherwise. The problem is that of the unavoidable necessity of thinking within the very structures which we seek to contest (Derrida 1981b), and that the task of deconstruction is to demonstrate the inherent instability of those same concepts which we must perforce go on using. This is what Spivak means when she refers to deconstruction as a 'critique of something that is extremely useful, something without which we cannot do anything' (1989b: 129).

To think the subject and subjectivity differently is most certainly to give up on the unified, self-present and pre-given subject of modernity, but it need not suggest a permanent state of fragmentation. Contrary to certain construals of postmodernism – and it should always be remembered that that term cannot itself represent any coherent whole – what I understand the deconstruction of the subject to entail is its constant re-formation in specific, local and temporary configurations. The claim is not simply that the contexts of subjectivity are multifarious and kaleidoscopic, but that, given there is no prior subject as such, then the positions occupied in themselves construct subjectivity as diverse and provisional. And these subject positions may correspond to what Foucault characterises as social vacancies (1972: 95–6). I do not, however, believe that an understanding of the subject as that which is constantly reconstituted need imply either that it is wholly indeterminate, or alternately that its construction is deterministic. It does not require a foundational subject to make sense of the concept of resistance, nor to belie the charge of passivity. And moreover, in parallel to the way that Butler marks the relationship between 'sex' and regulatory norms (1993: 2), the very fact that constitutive practices are reiterative indicates a persistent failure to achieve closure, to overcome resistance. The Deleuzean notion of desire as that which eludes co-option by the forces of the social might seem to offer a more creditable approach, but it should be remembered that Foucault himself had already characterised desire as both product and productive. The complex interplay of power and resistance is central to an analytics of the subject.

What seems clear – and this has surely been wrongly posed as a dilemma for feminism – is that we cannot continue to speak of subjectivity in the conventional sense, but I do not see that as a loss for women. Some male postmodernists have happily or perhaps cynically abandoned the subject altogether, or else, like the earlier Derrida with his 'incalculable choreographies', have treated the notion more as a matter of deconstructive play. As women, having been denied recognition all along, we cannot afford to dismiss ourselves so lightly, to allow ourselves to be without anchors in a situation in which existing power differentials, now theoretically detached from old forms but uncontested by new forms of subjectivity, will surely attach themselves to other points of reference. It seems to me crucial therefore that we should have a proper, albeit celebratory, place for subject positions within feminist theory, perhaps in the nomadic sense envisaged by Deleuze and provisionally endorsed by Braidotti (1991a), but clearly as the focus of the valorisation of women as moral agents. What is irrecuperable is the stability of the transcendental 'I', for although the fiction of identity over time is an appealing one, it must be continually questioned in order to keep open the discursive space of possibility. Far from destroying the notion of agency, the deconstruction of the subject forces us to recognise the plurality of its possibilities.

Several points need to be stressed here. First, the volatility of subject positions should not preclude us from taking a stand at any given strategic moment, nor from forming provisional coalitions of like interests. Second, the recognition that the humanist subject is discursively constructed, but never fully determined, by a nexus of exclusionary practices should allow us to resignify the parameters of agency. Instead of foreclosure on who may and who may not be classed as a (moral) agent, postmodernism – at least as it is appropriated by feminism – opens up the possibility of intervention from those places that have hitherto been fixed and marginalised. And it is an intervention not into pre-existing structures of power, but into the very processes of power which construct some of us as permanent others. Finally, the issue is not to block differentiation entirely, but to suspend its sedimentation. What I am suggesting is that the ethical moment consists not in the exercise of moral agency grounded on an as-if and necessary moment of definition, but in the very movement of *différance*. And what distinguishes it as ethical, in what I take to be the primary sense that precedes the morality of codes, is the acknowledgement that the values to be expressed might be otherwise.

The point I am making is that, despite the specific focus of the feminist project on valorising women, the move towards subject positions has wider implications. It goes much further than the very understandable desire on the part of some theorists to achieve that end solely in the sense of overturning, reversing the dominant hierarchical relations of patriarchy; and moreover it rejects the notion of a unified and enduring subject. The female move from margins to centre, and the repositioning of men as others, has, as I have already said, a provisional strategic appeal, but it is clearly inappropriate as a final goal. One problem is that the very relations of sameness and difference which, as we saw earlier, guarantee the patriarchal order, are left intact. Both the type of radical feminism expounded by Mary Daly (1979), with her clear call for new women-centred relations of power – or even for separatism – based on a kind of essential female energy, and the maternal thinking proposed by Sara Ruddick (1990a) with its stress on the superior caring nature of women, are implicated in such a charge. In addition, neither model goes beyond the human-ist presupposition of an integrated subjectivity, but simply seeks to substitute new affectional markers for the old abstract ones.

The attempt to define women's subjectivity in opposition to the masculine is seductive but ultimately self-defeating. Simply to reallocate the differential discursive power between the sexes is to fail to challenge the very basis on which liberal humanism oper-ates, and to leave open the possibility that the hierarchy will once more be reversed. And even were the enduring stability of such a female subjectivity guaranteed, its foundation on difference and exclusion would reiterate the very qualities which have disquali-fied not just women, but all the other others, in the first place. As such it could not meet my primary criterion for a feminist ethic, that of respect for differences as irreducibly plural and non-assimilable. What is needed if the feminist project is ever to be realised is that it should situate itself in the disintegration of oppo-sitional differences so that the relations of power which have sustained the patriarchy can no longer be reproduced, albeit in an obverse form. But this is not yet to deny sexual difference, and indeed I see a revision of the meaning of the term as crucial to the positioning of women as subjects in our own right. As Luce Irigaray explains it, the task is to 'secure a place for the feminine within sexual difference'. She goes on:

> That difference – masculine/feminine – has always operated 'within' systems that are representative, self-representative, of the (masculine) subject. . . . [O]ne sex and its lack, its atrophy, its negative, still does not add up to two. In other words, the feminine has never been defined except as the inverse, indeed the underside, of the masculine. So for woman it is not a matter of installing herself within this lack, this negative, even by denouncing it, nor of reversing the economy of sameness by turning the feminine into *the standard for 'sexual difference'*; it is rather a matter of trying to practice that difference.
>
> (1985b: 159)

Despite what Irigaray seems to suggest elsewhere, I suspect that the aim of a complete dismantlement of the apparatus, both discursive and non-discursive, of oppression must remain Utopian. Spivak, for example, takes a more realistic approach when she emphasises the importance of negotiation with male violence (1989a: 209; 1990: 147), or with the structures of Western liberalism: 'one tries to change something one is obliged to inhabit, since one is not writing from the outside. In order to keep one's effectiveness, one must also preserve those structures, not cut them down completely' (1990: 72). What may be possible is a radical and thorough displacement of the configuration of power relations and a reconstruction that constitutes difference not as binary opposites but as reconcilable diversities. The liberal humanist conception of difference, the difference that in fact sustains the economy of the same, the ubiquitous reference to the single masculine standard, would give way to an acknowledgement of differences as expressed in the specificity and multiplicity of both sexes.

It may be objected here that although I have consistently identified sameness and difference as being at the heart of the failed liberal humanist project, I have nevertheless, in my references to specificity and in agreement with Irigaray as above, taken as given the difference between women and men, albeit as a very different form of sexual difference. But far from setting up a conflict of approach, in an important sense I see the move as required by not just the feminist but the poststructuralist agenda. Indeed, to do otherwise would be to reinstate the standard of sameness, to re-enact the kind of gender indifference that underlies the notion of the universal subject. And yet it is not the insistence on difference as such that informs the poststructuralist feminist agenda so much as the multiplicity of differences, and these of course will include those of ethnicity, class, sexuality and so on as well as gender. Women do not stand in opposition to men in some kind of either/or struggle for subjectivity; the task is to recognise *all* the others and acknowledge their *inclusiveness* in the construction of the gendered self. The starting point for the affirmation of ourselves as subjects of our own discourse lies not in constructing yet another counter-identity but in insisting on the radical plurality, particularity and provisionality of all discourses. Nonetheless, gender is an important analytic category here and now, and I would argue further that even if the relations of power were to be sufficiently displaced so that sexual oppression were no longer the reality of women's everyday lives, sexual difference would remain as an irreducible element in the construction of the subject. It is not that I wish to take biology as determinate – and in any case biological knowledge comes to us as always already mediated by discourse – but to emphasise that the denial of sexual difference suppresses how it is, specifically, to become a subject in a body defined as female.

SEXUAL DIFFERENCE

Before taking up the issue of what relevance embodiment might have to a feminist rewriting of the subject, I want to turn in more depth to the question of sexual difference, for it is here perhaps that the feminist poststructuralist agenda diverges most markedly from the path mapped out by the male surveyors of the post-modern. The problem that we must resolve is that if the binary sexual difference of masculine/feminine is displaced, then what grounds could there be for seeking a political and ethical position for women *per se*? What would it mean for sexual differentials to survive the deconstruction of the binary? The underlying question of whether or not an ethics can be gender-neutral must concern itself too with the tension between singularity and universality, and with the postmodernist claim to dissolve all universal categories. What I shall be suggesting is that it is precisely the embodied specificity of sexual difference that takes it beyond the epistemology of the binary and grounds it as an irreducible component of feminist ethics.

It is not immediately clear that sexual difference *can* retain a place as an analytic category, and much recent feminist theory has been obliged to reintroduce it simply as a strategic necessity. Now there is nothing wrong with that so long as the expediency of the move is recognised – as it always is by Spivak, for example (1988: 77) – and the task of contesting the discursive supports of phallogocentrism continues unabated. In this sense the 'as-if' of the feminine serves as a point of departure only, a provisional and temporary ontology from which to launch the raids on male epistemology which will eventually collapse its own position. This seems to me very different from the type of feminine stand-point, theorised initially by Hartsock (1983), which entirely fails to problematise the subject of oppression, but simply takes for granted its unified though marginal integrity. Standpoint theory has been much criticised both explicitly and implicitly, particularly by black feminists, for its exclusions (Lorde 1984; Martin and Mohanty 1988; Spelman 1990); but it is not clear that a greater sensitivity to issues of race, class, age, sexuality and so on does more than diversify the grounds on which a stand is made. In postmodernist theory, specificity *alone* is not enough, for it fails to challenge the assumption that the one who knows precedes that which is known.

In contrast to this modified form of humanism, Donna Haraway's iconoclastic 'Manifesto for cyborgs' (1990) seems to dissolve the boundaries of the subject completely, and though she speaks for feminism, it is doubtful that sexual difference has any purchase in her brave new world.[6] The cyborg is neither woman nor even human, but a fabricated hybrid of 'machine and organism' which cuts through the discrete categories which constitute our differences as women:

> There is nothing about being 'female' that naturally binds women. There is not even such a state as 'being' female, itself a highly complex category constructed in contested sexual scientific discourses and other social practices. Gender, race, or class consciousness is an achievement forced on us by the terrible historical experience of the contradictory social realities of patriarchy, colonialism, racism, and capitalism.
>
> (Haraway 1990: 197).

Though she does not cite him, Haraway's materialist concerns are clearly nearer to Foucault than to Derrida; and in the absence of a totalising theory of sexual difference, she puts emphasis on the local and partial configurations through which women may challenge their oppressions. The cyborg speaks to 'an intimate experience of boundaries' (1990: 223), but not as the outcome of rigidly prescribed limits, but as a consequence of flux and transformation. The 'Manifesto' provides a highly evocative vision of feminist politics in a technological age, a vision which engages as much with the cultural postmodernity associated with Baudrillard as with the implications of 'philosophical' postmodernism. For a more abstract insight into the fate of sexual difference within a reconceived philosophical field, we must turn elsewhere.

I have indicated already that Irigaray is one of those who embraces the initial stages of poststructuralist analysis and yet retains a place for the feminine, which she intends as a resistant move. On an explicit level, her heretical stance is most clearly directed at traditional and Lacanian psychoanalysis, where the boundaries of sexual difference are defined by reference to the presence or absence of the penis/phallus. In contrast, the notion of the feminine that Irigaray seeks to bring into being rejects the relation to the transcendental signifier and looks to the imaginary female body as the ground for a reconceived Symbolic. What more concerns me here, however, is the way in which Irigaray's work implicitly engages with and throws into focus the limitations of Derrida's approach to sexual difference. While it is generally the case that Derrida has written very little on the particularity of women, his whole project of deconstruction must inevitably recast sexual difference. Like Lacan, Derrida would reject a biological ground for fixed gender differences, but he would go further in showing that if gender is constituted in language then it cannot effect the closure that Lacan seems to imply, but must be open always to resignification. It is not, however, a reinterpretation that will satisfy Irigaray.

We may begin to discern the nature of Derrida's engagement with the feminine in *Spurs: Nietzsche's Styles* (1979) where he teases out Nietzsche's three positions on the 'woman question'. Of these – woman as non-truth; as truth; and as the non-truth of truth – Derrida appears to align himself provisionally with the last. And it is that concept of undecidability that becomes the privileged marker for woman in subsequent Derridean texts in which the metaphorical 'feminine' underwrites the deconstruction of the logos. It is an appropriation that has alarmed many feminists (Jardine 1985; de Lauretis 1987), though I should want to stress that in giving a poststructuralist account, Derrida cannot, in his own terms, lay claim to represent the one true way. Nevertheless it is instructive to address Derrida's specific attempts, particularly in the 1982 interview published as 'Choreographies',[7] to engage with and rewrite sexual difference. What I shall suggest is that the position he adopts may be incompatible not simply with the type of deconstructive feminist agenda, exemplified by Luce Irigaray, that wants to write women back into the symbolic as *radically different*, but with Derrida's own move towards an ethical concern with the otherness of the other.

In 'Choreographies' Derrida fills out some of his earlier references to the feminine and to feminism, and offers what seems to
me a fairly sympathetic reading of the tension between the
necessity for political action on behalf of women as an oppressed
group, and a kind of maverick feminism which exceeds oppositional sexual difference to enter into a multiplicity of sexual
differences. The distinction that is drawn is between a reactive
form of feminism, which corresponds to the term as derided by
Nietzsche – and indeed, despite disclaimers, by some Derridean
texts[8] – and one which is endorsed as a Utopian dream where the
dreamer is Derrida himself. Unlike many feminist critics – Rosi
Braidotti, for example, pointedly writes such male-endorsed feminism as 'pheminism' (1987: 233) – I do not see Derrida's remarks
as antagonistic to the real life, everyday struggles of women, so
much as cautionary against making those the sole focus for
women. And indeed any of us who are engaged in theorising a
poststructuralist response to patriarchal power must necessarily
value the creation of discursive spaces in which to rethink sexual
difference. But yet I remain uneasy that the polysexual signatures
of the dance – Derrida's playful metaphor for the pluralised
subject positions beyond gender – might not preclude important
feminist and ethical considerations. When Derrida dreams that
the differences will be 'sexual otherwise' (1985a, 'Choreographies':
184), what does he really mean?

As I understand it, his initial step is a clearing operation which
analyses sexual difference in two forms, both of which are trapped
within a phallogocentric discourse. The first and by now familiar
form, and the one against which traditional (and in Nietzschean
terms reactive) feminism has implicitly set itself, is the oppositional binary of masculine/feminine in which difference marks the
inferiority of the second term *in relation* to the primary referent.
In other words, what is set up is an hierarchical structure of difference which collapses into the economy of the same where women
are always the absent presence. As Derrida explains: 'The determination of sexual difference in opposition is destined, designed,
in truth, for truth; it is so in order to erase sexual difference'
(1985a, 'Choreographies': 175). At its limit, the Hegelian dialectic
fails to deliver a new third term, and any feminist appropriation
of power which neglects to challenge the model itself does no
more than reverse the hierarchy without disturbing its economy.
It is the same point that Irigaray consistently makes.

In his highly condensed references to Heidegger and Levinas, Derrida considers a second mode of sexual difference in which a supposedly neutral ontology precedes the sexual marking of the binary. 'Choreographies' itself does not make clear the danger of the Heideggerian approach, but in another work Derrida suggests that Heidegger's explicit exclusion of sexual difference might represent an operation of violence (1991a, 'Geschlecht': 390). In a similar way, the attempt by Levinas to posit an originary humanity before the sexual division founders on his marking of the initial status of the pre-differential as masculine, and sexual difference itself as femininity. Far from empowering an ethics, as Derrida glosses it, as 'that relationship to the other as other which accounts for no other determination or sexual characteristic in particular' (1985a, 'Choreographies': 178), the ethical project of Levinas results, as Gayatri Spivak tersely remarks in another context – though Derrida merely signals a slight unease – in a 'prurient heterosexist, male-identified ethics' (Spivak 1992: 77). Nonetheless, the question has been raised that if ontological neutrality cannot precede sexuality, then might not there be another sexual difference, an irreducible difference *before* the two?

The floor is cleared then for Derrida's own dance with the poly-sexual signatures, those markers of plurality, of sexual differences, and of an irreducible dissymmetry which he evokes and likens in 'Choreographies' to 'a kind of reciprocal, respective and respectful excessiveness' (1985a: 184). This seems to me a tempting way of grounding an ethics of difference as one which can celebrate singularity without the fetish of an essential subject of truth as such. But one issue remains unanswered here which may yet unsettle the approbation of postmodernist feminists. Without wanting to assign a temporal meaning to the question, it is this: is the sexual-otherwise thought 'before', taking off 'from', or 'within' sexual difference in the conventional binary sense? On the Heideggerian model proposed above, it is difficult to avoid the double sense of priority, and equally perhaps the inevitability of the arrest of multiplication in binary sexual difference; whereas at the end of 'Choreographies' Derrida has seemed to favour another way when he asks: 'what if we were to reach, what if we were to approach here (for one does not arrive at this as one would at a determined location) the area of a relationship to the other where the code of sexual marks would no longer be discriminating?'

(1985a: 184). In either case binary sexual difference is displaced and superseded; but displaced, note, without the thought of an other sexual difference no longer positioned as a hierarchy, an other difference in which, exceeding the economy of the same, the female term might really be other *than* the male.

Now, given that a rigid gender hierarchy is precisely what is at issue for feminism whether that is characterised as reactive or deconstructive – and I am by no means certain that such a distinction could or should be made – the type of move made by Derrida might seem wholly to be welcomed. Nonetheless it is not the only possible response, nor, even, I shall argue the most ethically appropriate one. Where the Derrida of 'Choreographies' would have each of us as polysexual in interaction with polysexual others, one alternative is that, from within the oppositional sexual difference which we experience now, the feminine should be recuperated as distinctively other, rather than as more of the same. In other words, if sexual difference now is predicated on a single referent, the male, then could 'sexual otherwise' indicate what Luce Irigaray would call 'the other of the other'? In contradistinction to the explicit Lacanian denial of that notion, it is Irigaray's contention that women are the necessary but excluded ground of the symbolic, marked only as the other *of* men, thus incorporated within the same, or else wholly excessive and silenced.[9] Within the Symbolic women function as the mirror whose surface confirms the self-reflection, self-presence of men without itself being represented. Indeed, in so far as they are recognised at all, it is as objects, or as Irigaray puts it as 'commodities' used and exchanged by men: 'The use, consumption and circulation of their sexualized bodies underwrites the organisation and reproduction of the social order in which they have never taken part as "subjects"' (1985b: 84). Sexual difference functions then only in the limiting sense that the visibility of women is the visibility of the mother alone, as object, and of the daughter who will supplant her. There is no other possible position for women, only exclusion. Her strategy therefore is to give voice to the feminine as radically other within a reconceived symbolic which re-cognises the mother-other, mother-matter, other-lover (1985b: *passim*). For her, rather than the displacement of sexual difference, it is precisely the recovery/discovery of it – as the place where wonder ('*admiration*') might mediate the gap between man and woman – that is the crucial issue. Irigaray, then, calls for a sexual difference that has never yet existed between the sexes, one where: 'wonder maintains their autonomy within their statutory difference, keeping a space of freedom and attraction between them, a possibility of separation and alliance' (1993a: 13). It is a project to give place to both the sexed and the material, and one which seems to me inherently ethical in its opening up of the closure of the binary.

In common with Irigaray, Derrida has charted the simultaneous capture and evasion of women within the logos, but he puts his emphasis on displacement, always insisting that the catachrestic signifier 'Woman' is the undecidable, subversive force which splits open the logic of the binary from the inside. This highly metaphorical Woman is that which disrupts the metaphysics of presence: 'that which will not be pinned down by truth is, in truth – feminine' (Derrida 1979: 55). She is the veil of the text, writing itself, which stripped aside reveals only the Nietzschean non-truth of truth. She is like the supplement, *différance*, the trace, the hymen – that privileged figure of undecidability, both inside and outside, virginity and marriage at once (1981a, *Dissemination*). This promiscuous feminisation of the otherness within elicits growing doubts as to its compatibility with the feminist agenda, for as Lois McNay writes: 'it is not clear to what extent the supposedly radical equation of woman with that which cannot be contained within discourse is very different from traditional stereotypes of woman as unknowable and unrepresentable' (1992: 17). For Derrida, Woman is everything incalculable; everything, that is, but the bearer of such 'essentializing fetishes' as female sexuality. And that, I would contend, is the point of rupture, where even postmodernist feminists might say 'enough'. We also want to operate in the textual spaces, want to overflow the restrictive stereotypes of femininity, want to exploit the leakiness of the logos, yet not at the expense of female sexuality, but because of it. We write in white ink, and we also bleed.[10] The endless metaphors of Woman may serve some discursive purpose, but if we are to enter into the ethical and political, then it is my contention that we must insist on the materiality of women's bodies, and on the specificity of our sexual otherness.

For all the concentration on the displacement and undecidability of the feminine it is in any case unlikely that Derrida means by that that the feminine is indeterminate. Certainly in the 'After-word' to *Limited Inc*, subtitled 'Toward an ethic of discussion', in a discussion of interpretation in general, he writes: 'I want to recall that undecidability is always a *determinate* oscillation between possibilities', and again, '[t]here would be no indecision or *double bind* were it not between *determined* (semantic, ethical, political) poles, which are upon occasion terribly necessary and always irreplaceably singular' (1988: 148). The implication, if I can carry it over into the present discussion, is that the undecidable feminine nevertheless operates within the parameters of a sexual difference which may itself be a necessary reality. But there is a further consideration, namely that the undecidability of women, as Derrida indicates in the seminar published as 'Women in the beehive' (1987: 181–204), may be of at least two different types. The first, which is of the type outlined above, is that which falls within the structural economy of binary sexual difference, within the order of the calculable, 'a kind of programming or unprogramming a program' (1987: 195). The second is excessive to that calculus, and may correspond to that undecidability that paradoxically is named in *Limited Inc* as the necessary condition 'for decision in the order of ethical-political responsibility'(1988: 116). It is not clear whether one can speak of Woman in the second mode, but the points that Derrida makes, and which I want to stress, are that the relationship between modes is not necessarily chronological, and that undecidability is never complete. The radical incalculability of women is just that, rooted; and rooted I would suggest in the always already of the sexed body whose gender is not mapped by biology.

Feminist deconstructionists have no difficulty in agreeing that there is no one place for woman, but would reject the implication, as Derrida suggests provocatively in 'Choreographies', that there is no place at all (1985a: 168). His response would be, perhaps, that *Woman* must be everywhere, but that is a very different vision from the widely accepted feminist 'demand' that *women* should be everywhere. The outline that Derrida gives of the necessity for woman to 'challenge a certain idea of the locus and the place' (ibid.) is uncontroversial; but what are we to make of his appeal to 'this indeterminable number of blended voices, this mobile of non-identified sexual marks whose choreography can carry, divide, multiply the body of each "individual"' (1985a: 184)? Given that Derrida explicitly rejects any 'new' concept of woman (1985a: 174), then should we not be wary that at the limit the dream of everywhere may dissolve into nowhere? In a powerful defence of his position, Drucilla Cornell suggests that Derrida's intention is to avoid making for women a new proper place, and making of them a new object of knowledge (Cornell 1991: 86), but she sees too the need for the affirmation of the feminine before the polysexuality of the dance. Where I cannot agree with her is in the contention that 'the choreographic text still involves designatable masculine and feminine voices' (1991: 93). Could it not be that the 'blended voices' that Derrida privileges in 'Choreographies' indicate not a new kind of sexual difference beyond the binary, but the annihilation of sexual/textual distinctions? Is not the image of the polysexual multiple choreographies of the dance a dream of absolute indistinction, the last chance perhaps for the threatened ontology of the masculine to reinscribe itself in the guise of the undecidable? Faced with the move directly from a discourse in which women are defined either as the other of the same, or as the unspoken and unspeaking slippage of the gender binary, to a discourse of 'blended' voices, I cannot but wonder what is to stop the old familiar generic 'he' from occupying the places of enunciation. Though Derrida's deconstructive approach has consistently disturbed a structuralist model of language which knows no other of the other, and though he himself may resist offering a new representation of women, the space that he ostensibly vacates, the space that is that opens up to the Utopian dream of the dance, may yet fail to realise the voices of women, as other of the other. Indeed, while the material relationships of power between men and women remain relatively undisturbed, and until masculinity itself is divested of the privilege of speaking and naming, it is difficult to see why women should accede to Derrida's dream.

I am by no means suggesting that women can afford to ignore the incalculable choreographies of the dance, or should run the risk of reifying sexual difference in a simple reversal of the oppositional structure. If the failure of traditional ethics to be adequate to women can be located in the complementary moves of either claiming the sexual neutrality of the ethical or of marginalising the female as the marked term of the sexual binary, then clearly the move beyond simple difference must be an ethical project. Indeed, to remain always within the calculable is to remain within the economy of the same, which as Derrida has made clear – in the 'Afterword' to *Limited Inc* (1988), and in 'Eating well' (1991b), for example – marks the impossibility of ethics. Nonetheless, in the light of his more recent work on what, in his 1991 Amnesty lecture, he called the ethics of affirmation, which demands an openness to differences, I am not sure how far Derrida would want now to endorse 'blended voices'.[11] If ethical responsibility lies in the obligation to 'protect the other's otherness' (Derrida 1991b: 111), is that not also a call for sexual specificity, which is in turn incompatible with blended voices? As I understand it, it is the irreducible alterity of the other which grounds both address and response, the call to the self, which is the precondition of ethical discourse. If what is at issue for women are those phallogocentric strategies which reify us within the same, then surely ethical responsibility demands openness to the sexual otherwise as the sexual other. And for the project of feminism as resistance, it is not only, as Spivak says (1988: 77), that definitions are necessary to allow us to make a stand, but also that women must take the space within which to construct our own metaphors, to speak an irreducible sexual difference from which to shatter the closure of the gender binary. And that is where Derrida's analysis diverges most clearly from the agenda that Irigaray sets herself. While both may want to facilitate the attempt to disrupt the univocal nature of language so that the masculine, in Irigaray's words, 'could no longer, all by itself, define, circumvene, circumscribe, the properties of any thing and everything' (1985b: 80), she alone is committed to the reconstitution of the feminine in its sexual specificity.

EMBODYING THE SUBJECT

Throughout the previous section it will have become apparent that in contradistinction to the disembodied play of differences which concern Derrida, I favour a feminist rewriting of the subject that demands an attention to the corporeal body. Now this sense of embodiment is precisely what has been omitted most often from masculine accounts of subjectivity. One major point of the post-Cartesian notion of the universal, transcendent subject is that *he* is constituted in the radical separation of mind from body. The privileging of the so-called higher faculties of reason, intellect, spirit and so on over the material and mundane grounds a two-tier system in which women, tied as they ostensibly are to their bodies, and most particularly to their reproductive bodies, have been deemed largely incapable of autonomous rational thought.

Quite simply, women are deemed to live their bodies in ways that men are not, and this constraint on transcendence is alone sufficient to disqualify them from full subjectivity. The absent body characterises male/moral discourse, and women, being all too solid, are paradoxically situated in that absence. If, then, women are to occupy subject positions not by reiterating the split and practising transcendence, but by reclaiming the unity of body and mind, then we must do so by affirming embodiment. Nancy Fraser has seen the 'rhetoric of bodies and pleasures' as a useful tactical device (1989: 62), but it is surely more complex than just another oppositional move. It has, I think, a great deal more to offer than a reactive feminism, such as that which would embrace an identity between women in/as their bodies and the forces of nature, in either a material or spiritual sense (Daly 1979; Griffin 1980). The point rather is to displace the convention and break the link between subject positions and exclusion, whether that exclusion is of the female or of the corporeal.

With that in mind, it is important to mark here that yet again the specific devaluation of the female element in moral discourse, indeed the denial of female subjectivity, is mirrored in the often unexpressed but very real devaluation of those who are sick. Although the usual phenomenological understanding of sickness sees it in terms of the 'broken' body, that should not be taken to imply that the whole body is an integral feature of subjectivity. It may be the necessary ground – one is reminded here of Irigaray's notion of the place of the suppressed feminine in masculine discourse – but it is not overtly present to the experiencing subject. The broken body, however, demands attention, and sickness becomes highly stressful to self-identity: 'The fidelity of our bodies is so basic that we never think of it – it is the certain grounds of our daily experience. Chronic illness is a betrayal of that fundamental trust. We feel under siege' (Kleinman 1988: 45). In the light of this, Kleinman goes on to suggest that the physician's task should be to encourage narratives of embodiment. In reality, of course, the intervention of health-care professionals may be directed in quite another way: rather than the reincorporation of the self, what is aimed at is the restoration of the healthy body as the body that is forgotten *and* transcended. This split between body and self becomes clearer in the formulation proposed by Drew Leder in *The Absent Body* (1990), in which he characterises the experience of ill health as 'the absence of an absence'. In common with Kleinman, it is Leder's contention that in the normal course of events, the body is scarcely experienced phenomenologically at all. In other words, as long as it gives no cause for concern it is not consistently present to us, but once the body falls sick, or becomes 'broken', then it forces itself into our consciousness and that comfortable absence is lost. But that new awareness is not integrated into the sense of self; rather, the body is perceived, but remains other: 'The body is no longer alien-as-forgotten, but precisely as-remembered, a sharp and searing presence threatening the self' (Leder 1990: 91).

This state of what Leder calls dys-appearance can result both from the dysfunctional nature of ill health, and in the more Sartrean social sense, as a result of the everyday objectifying gaze of another.[12] In either case it is experienced as a denial of subjectivity, and must result, one infers, in embodiment being associated symbolically with disruption. If Leder is correct in his analysis, then clearly the situation in which patients can typically find themselves in a power relationship with health-care professionals, where they experience their bodies as both 'broken' and the object of scrutiny, heavily reinforces the ontological devaluation of embodiment. As Ros Diprose points out, however, there is a problem with Leder's model of ill health in that 'the disruption to the texture of the self which occurs when the body's integrity is altered' (Diprose 1994: 111) is not – as he seems to infer – necessarily negative nor coincident with 'brokenness'. And what concerns me further here is that those things which for women constitute the usual lifelong and continuous capacities of, and changes to, the body – such as puberty, menstruation, reproduction, lactation or menopause – are characteristically posed nevertheless as medical problems. Leder acknowledges Iris Young's claim that it is only middle-aged men[13] who really see their bodies as unchanging (Leder 1990: 88), but he fails to note that it is female body events that are habitually the site of clinical intervention. The universalised, and more or less quiescent, body of phenomenology is essentially male and healthy, and the subjectivity that is defined over and against that body is a highly normative construct. In consequence, the inescapable and distinctive embodiment of those persons deemed to be in less than normative health becomes a determinant of their being treated as less than full subjects, as less than capable of independent moral agency.

It is notable that despite his rewriting of the phenomenology of ill health, and a passing awareness of its gender limitations, Leder reiterates the masculine bias of that discourse in assuming that the 'experience' of corporeal absence is common to all. His explanation of the devaluation of the body, as it relates to the experience of sickness, may reflect cultural mores, but it leaves unaddressed other more gender-specific determinants. It is at least arguable that women – and indeed children, adolescents and older people – experience their bodies as a continuing presence, rarely entirely forgotten, and that that experience may be both positive and negative. That so many 'healthy' changes to the female body are nevertheless brought under medical control, and that matters such as weight, comportment and appearance are the object of intense scrutiny, speaks to a deep cultural unease with the embodiment of women. Moreover, the inherent threat of internal disruption in sickness is paralleled by the ever-present reality of potentially hostile external intervention into their body spaces, and into the space of their bodies. The relationship between the (broken) body as other and the feminine as other, both in relation to the masculine subject, is a highly complex one, and suggests again that those defined as sick are en-gendered as female. What both seem to encompass is the paradox that what is devalued is also the most threatening.

A similar paradox, though couched in somewhat different terms, marks twentieth-century psychoanalysis, which despite the impetus it has given to the deconstruction of the unified subject is nevertheless, like clinical medicine, marked by the distinctive mind/body split at the heart of philosophical modernity. In the poststructuralist take-up of Freud, the recovery of the notion of the unconscious is shown to initiate two things:

1 it fundamentally challenges the fixed certainties of the masculine rational subject authorised by his own discourse, a discourse in which, as Irigaray puts it, '[l]icense to operate is only granted to the (so-called) play of those differences that are measured in terms of *sameness*' (1985a: 247); and
2 in so far as the feminine eludes the economy of the same, it yet further relegates women as being the dark continent beyond representation, as being outside of discourse altogether. In Lacanian terms, when the man or rather male child enters the Symbolic, the arena of language use, he both constructs and

confirms his superiority in an identification with the Name of the Father, while the woman remains other, unable to assimilate to a language not her own, and tied to the pre-Oedipal Imaginary. And that paradigmatically is the realm of indifferentiation, not between male and female in this case, but between mother and child.

Women then are neither fully autonomous nor authentic language users, but are irrecoverably set in the pre-discursive body. And that body as such is effectively the absent body.

Clearly, such a limited précis does little justice to the complexities of the relevant psychoanalytic theory, nor to the numerous feminist challenges and modifications to it, but it does make my point that the embodiment of women, however it is characterised, is consistently treated as a feature to be set against the successful tenure or construction of subjectivity. In counterpart to the Renaissance and post-Enlightenment understanding of the immanence of the leaky female body, Lacanian theory has it as both excessive and absent. In *Seminar XX, Encore* Lacan declares: 'There is a *jouissance* proper to her, to this "her" which does not exist and which signifies nothing' (Mitchell and Rose 1982: 145). And in a notorious aside he points to Bernini's statue of the ecstatic St Teresa as, presumably, an example of a body that overflows itself and yet remains beyond the bounds of signification. The move that Lacan makes, to somehow reify the feminine without giving it any texturality, is familiar in much poststructuralist and postmodernist theory. The abstraction of Woman as the repository of all that exceeds the logos (as, for example, in 'the non-truth of truth'), and as a refuge from the Law of the Father, seems to have little or nothing to do with the concrete experiences and aspirations of 'real' women. Where the feminine is taken to represent all that is other than the logic of the binary – a binary, that is, which is shown by poststructuralism to rest on the economy of the same – it may be accorded some reverence, but only in so far as it seems to be open to occupation by all those who would contest the conventional paradigms of ontology and epistemology. But that occupation is highly abstract and idealised, and above all leaves no place for bodily materiality, least of all that of women. When Deleuze, for example, uses the signifier of the 'becoming-woman', he refers not simply to the ongoing process of inscription on a Body-without-Organs, but to a body that is sexually undifferentiated (Braidotti 1991a: 116). In contrast, what has seemed important to many feminist postmodernists is that the body that becomes as it is inscribed has substance as well as surface, and moreover is always lived as sexed. It is not that there is any wish to reclaim the feminine as an essentialist quality, or even to mark it as belonging only to women, but to resist a male-authored recuperation of the feminine that either reiterates its incalculable otherness or occludes the sexed specificity of the body.

For that very reason then, postmodern feminist theory, in its project to integrate the excluded without losing touch with specificity, places new emphasis on reclaiming the body in both its corporeality and its desires, as the site of multiple subject positions. In other words, subjectivity is not simply dispersed and pluralised but nonetheless remains expressed in consciousness alone, becoming rather a matter of both style and substance. And the way in which women will construct and occupy those subject positions, what Spivak calls the 'I'-slots (1988: 243), will reflect both their particularity as embodied individuals and their generality as a sex. Inevitably the feminist re-presentation of the insights of postmodernism regarding the body will have significant implications for the issue of health care, and in turn for bioethics. Indeed, I would argue, along with Diprose (1994: 19), that any feminist ethics of health care must thematise not just embodiment, but differential embodiment from the start. Moreover, that move might uncover the way in which ethics, including the ethics of health care, is overdetermined by the specular at the expense of touch. The humanist moral self who acts and towards whom we have responsibilities is given as individual, clear-sighted, autonomous and unitary, both affirmed and threatened by the gaze of the other; in contrast, feminists might privilege a notion of contiguous bodies/selves touching and speaking together.

Before moving on, I shall recapitulate briefly. Despite its substantive area of enquiry, the traditional ethical model has been concerned primarily with the autonomous and disembodied individual where the primary focus has been the control and disposal of one's body as property. Given its reference back to the Cartesian split between mind and body in which the non-corporeal has been privileged as the site of subjectivity, it is an ethics that is out of touch with the body. What has concerned modernist ethics above all have been the abstract conditions for the interaction of pre-given, unified and rational subjects. The central question of bioethics – how should one act? – has appeared then to devolve on such issues as the potential conflict between interests, both individual/individual and individual/communal good, and has been mediated by principles of rights, equality, freedom, justice and so on. At the same time, in so far as the discipline of health care has functioned on the basis of normalisation, as Foucault has demonstrated, the effect of its restorative and curative practices may be characterised as reproducing a set of hierarchical binary differences. The bioethical body derives its significance, then, not as the site of my being in the world, but rather as the locus of relations of power between transcendent subjectivities. In contrast, the phenomenological account speaks to an integrated mind and body and does much to ground the subject in an everyday living out of the material body. The structure of the self is fully imbricated – albeit non-consciously – with its corporeal capacities, and moreover is constituted in its specificity by its engagement with external practices.

If, then, sickness represents a splitting between mind and body such that the one is estranged from, even threatened by, the other, then an ethics informed by the phenomenological model must be concerned with the restoration of an integrated self. What it fails to thematise, however, is the nature of the norms constituting that 'healthy' self, and in particular the way in which health-care practices themselves are not somehow outside the constitutive discourse but are important determinants in their own right. As my opening chapter in particular outlined, medicine and its related disciplines are never neutral or innocent, but are a central facet of the power/knowledge complex that constructs the appearance of a prior and privileged self. Moreover, as Foucault again has shown, attention to the individual functions simply in the service of a project of generalisation. Whether the dominant model is that of phenomenology or biomedicine, the universal nature of the healthy body operates to obscure the specificity of the particular bodies which either instantiate or elude its general claims. Differences are represented only in so far as they define the boundaries of the same.

As I have remarked before, the Foucauldian image of the body as the locus of external disciplinary practices draws together both discursive and material considerations. What constitutes

Foucault's field of enquiry are material signs, the manner in which the 'I', the subject of discourse is written on the body. It may be, of course, more subjected than subject, but what matters is its distance from the universal, transcendent 'I' of the *cogito*. Nonetheless, what his move suggests, or at least leaves open, is the lurking potential, more clearly evidenced in other postmodernist discourses, that if the body is simply the 'inscribed surface of events' then its substantiality will be flattened out to become in effect a blank page passively open to all and any inscription. While I do not in any way wish to deny the multiplicity of inscriptions, what is equally important for feminist postmodernism is the insistence that there is no singular mode of determination. The model of subjectivity proposed by Liz Grosz (1994) – as a Möbius strip which defies notions of inside and outside – is an attractive one, though I would want to treat with some caution her distinction between corporeal exteriority and psychical interiority. As I understand it, the corporeal itself is both surface text and in-depth substance, not in the sense of two separate component parts, nor even as a passive overlay of the one by the other. What is intended is the sense of interactive and mutually constituent modes of being. And moreover, although on the one hand the body, and the body as subject, may be read as a script in production, on the other that subject is always already embodied, and more particularly embodied as gendered.

Though several writers have shown a limited engagement with a postmodernist analysis of health-care issues (Armstrong 1983; Turner 1987, 1992; Braidotti 1989a, 1991b), and Diprose (1994) has developed an embodied ethics which can throw new light on biomedicial discourse, there has been, to date, very little sustained or consistent work done in the area. Even more unusual is any investigation of what a postmodernist health care itself might entail, and Nicholas Fox's text *Postmodernism, Sociology and Health* (1993) stands alone in turning towards that direction. Although notable for its attempt to move away from the sociological in order to investigate some of the ethical implications of a new approach, Fox's book is disappointing in that it reiterates the masculine trope of disembodiment by insisting on the distinction between the anatomical and the inscribed body. In any case Fox apparently fails to appreciate that the Deleuzean body-without-organs on which he relies 'has nothing whatsoever to do with the body itself' (Deleuze and Guattari 1984: 8), for Fox himself states: 'The body of inscription is not the organic body of medicine. *In place of* the anatomical body, the body of interest here is a non-organic, political surface: a *Body-without-Organs*' (1993: 36; my emphasis). In his own terms, however, given that Fox (mis)recognises the fabrication of both types of bodies, it is difficult to understand just what distinction he is making, or how he would account for those material processes of change such as growing older, giving birth or dying. Whatever inscription is offered of those things, however much meaning is deferred, it makes little sense to deny that something substantial has happened. Moreover, in following the Deleuzean move of suspending the constraints of space and time as well as of materiality, Fox is unable to see that there is anything distinctive about the being, or rather becoming, of the body that is 'known' as female. In consequence he has nothing to say about sexual difference in its radical, Irigarayan sense, and he lightly dismisses Cixous's *écriture féminine* – which she sees as writing the female body – as uncomfortably essentialist (Fox 1993: 153).

Now that charge of essentialism has been one of the major stumbling-blocks to any unproblematic acceptance of the concept of embodiment as being of positive value to feminist theory. The difficulty is particularly acute for postmodernists in so far as it appears to speak to a biologism which is firmly rejected. The idea that there could be anything fundamental and certain about the body, and moreover that it could be sexed from the start, seems to invite at least some turn towards biological determinism as an explanation for the devaluation of women. The strategic arguments against essentialism, and indeed any form of feminism which has attempted to base a politics on female nature, are well rehearsed and I shall not further pursue them here, but merely note that so forceful has been the rejection of the body in some critiques that it seems almost to entail a wholly unintended effacement of women themselves. For postmodernists, it is, in any case, rather more than a matter of strategic avoidance. What is at issue is an analytics which takes as its *sine qua non* a scepticism towards, and deconstruction of, all foundational claims. If there is nothing outside the text, nothing but the text, then the biological body, still less the sexed body, cannot be grasped as a prediscursive reality. Corporeality is just another construct, and sexual difference is no more stable than gender difference. The distinction that Fox makes between the anatomical and Deleuzean body is therefore a superficially understandable one within the context of postmodernism, but feminists have been increasingly reluctant to let it go at that. Rosi Braidotti, for example, despite her own empathy with Deleuze, calls on 'the political will to assert the specificity of the lived, female bodily experience, the refusal to disembody sexual difference into a new allegedly postmodern anti-essentialist subject' (1989b: 91), and Ros Diprose (1994) is equally insistent both on the mutability of the phenomenonological body, and on an embodied and irreducible sexual difference.

The difficulty of squaring 'real' bodies with the deconstructionist approach is nowhere more apparent than in the response to the work of Luce Irigaray. What interests Irigaray is the way in which the inscription of femininity onto a female body is paralleled by the disembodiment of masculinity where disembodiment is consistently privileged. Given that she refers constantly to the anatomical differences between male and female, and she constructs an ontology and an ethics around just such differences, her supporters are constrained to explain how the claim against her of essentialism (Moi 1985; Sayers 1986; Weedon 1987) is misconstrued, or at very least overstated. One strategy, which is I think ultimately self-defeating, is to deny the physicality of the Irigarayan body and to posit it as purely textual (Grosz 1989: 111;[14] Berg 1991: 56); but that is to say that her project of prac-tising sexual difference is no less abstract than the masculine philosophy she critiques. The recuperation of the feminine as the other of the other clearly does involve finding a language, but it is a language in which to express the distinctive morphology of the female body, the two lips which differ in themselves and which are excessive to the isomorphic standard of the phallus. Moreover, although Irigaray certainly wants to operate within a reconceived Symbolic, the whole force of her deconstruction of the logos is that the latter is built on a denial of its material/maternal origins. In 'Plato's *Hystera*' (1985a), for example, she demonstrates that Descartes is just one point of reference in a long line of patriar-chal philosophy stretching back to Plato and beyond, in which the denial of corporeality in favour of the pure Intelligible/Idea repre-sents not just a male retreat from their own bodies, but a claim too to autogenesis. The Father-God, the ultimate arbiter, is relo-cated as the *source* of the Law, while the (m)other-matter is suppressed. But if Irigaray's gesture towards the corporeal is not simply a textual ploy, then is it after all essentialist?

A number of sympathetic commentators have suggested that Irigaray does indeed resort to essentialism, but that she does so in a strategic way. It is not that she really 'believes' in the reality of the female body, but that it provides a necessary referent for her reconception of the feminine as the excluded term of the masculine/feminine binary. Margaret Whitford (1991), for example, attempts to hold a delicate balance whereby Irigaray's perceived essentialism is a mimetic strategy aimed at resymbol-ising 'female' nature. But this too I think misses the point in that it accepts implicitly that essentialism and constructivism are opposed to each other. On the contrary, what Irigaray surely demonstrates is that such a putative opposition is just another binary which may be displaced by deconstruction. A similar view has been expressed by Gayatri Spivak (1989b) and Diana Fuss (1989), while Tina Chanter concludes that the charge of essen-tialism 'depends upon a variety of dichotomies that need to be questioned' (1995: 5).

An important part of Irigaray's strategy, then, is to interrupt the binary that positions the biological as static, ahistorical and determinate, and culture as representative of development and change. Against that convention, what her work stresses consistently is that culture also demands – indeed, depends on – constant repetition and sameness, while the biological is inher-ently interactive and dynamic. Although Irigaray may not satisfy some feminist demands for historical specificity, her project is centred, nonetheless, on writing the feminine into history and culture, and on recovering the morphology of a female body which is never one:

> When the/a woman touches herself ... a whole touches itself because it is infinite, because it has neither the knowledge nor the power to close up or to swell definitively to the extension of an infinite. This self-touching gives woman a form that is in(de)finitely transformed without closing over her appropria-tion. Metamorphoses occur in which there is no complete set, where no set theory of the One is established.
>
> (1985a: 233)

What concerns Irigaray above all, then, is to write in the suppressed physicality/desire of/for the body; but though she puts great emphasis, particularly in her later work, on the originary mother, it would be a mistake to see that as reduplicating the male symbolic move of recognising women only within the relations of (re)production. Far from endorsing an uncritical celebration of the place of the (m)Other, Irigaray has no wish to confine women to the prediscursive maternal body. The body towards which she gestures is determined by no one form. It is always plural, fluid and unbounded; a body that is not yet realised because not yet represented. It is then neither fixed nor solid nor singular, but it does have materiality and its possibilities are those of the distinctly feminine. On the horizons of becoming (what) matter(s) is reducible to neither essence nor text.[15]

The point that I want to emphasise here is that postmodernism need not be seen as tolerant only to the body that is conceived in wholly discursive terms, and neither need it accept a pre-given morphology as that on which inscription is simply overlaid. The flesh and blood givenness of the physical body is not a passive surface, but the site of sensation and libidinal desire which are in continuous interaction with textual practices. The female *jouissance* which overflows the closure of male discourse is not just an alternative linguistic construct, but an expression of a process of production at the interface of body, desire and language. The anatomical, social and discursive bodies are mutually constitutive, and none is complete in itself nor accessible independently of the other. And as with the ontology of the subject, the claim to epistemological certainty is just an illusion.

This type of deconstructionist approach which attempts to rethink the problems around essentialism and sexual difference represents a considerable move both from the radical indeterminacy of some postmodernism and from the liberal constructivist account. In that latter discourse, it is of course usual to distinguish sex from gender, so that while we may agree that gender is socially and discursively acquired, and may be sustained only through persistent recitation (Butler 1990, 1993), the implication is that sexed identity is a given. As I remarked in Chapter 1, Judith Butler outlines the view in *Gender Trouble* that gender is performative in terms of acts and gestures: '*performative* in the sense that the essence or identity that they otherwise purport to express are *fabrications* manufactured and sustained through corporeal signs and other discursive means' (1990: 136). But as a poststructuralist she is clear too that sex has no greater claim to be foundational and that the sex/gender binary split must be deconstructed. As I have argued earlier, and what I want to emphasise again, is that the meaning of the sexed body itself lies not in biological fact, but is constructed in and by representation.

It is not essentialist then to assert, and indeed I believe it would be deeply counterproductive as well as counter-intuitive to deny, that the experience of the body as sexed does situate, at very least, some attributes more firmly than others. In other words, there are consistent differences, though not essential ones, which have an effect. What is to be rejected is any implication that the sexed body predetermines *fixed* gender differences, or that the female subject can *only* speak the discourse of the other. I am on the contrary firmly committed to the idea that all gender signals can be radically displaced, though perhaps, and this is important, not all of them at once, and that subject positions are always fluid and provisional.

What can be drawn from the feminist enquiry into the lack of certainty about the subject, the rewriting of sexual difference, and the turn towards a positive sense of embodiment is the emergence of a celebratory form of femininity that insists on its difference. Far from erasing the intelligibility of the ethical, the postmodernist approach necessitates an ethic of openness and responsibility towards differences where none is given prior privilege. And those differences are not merely the external others, but the multiplicity of insistent differences within. Most radically, an acknowledgement of *différance* deconstructs any reliance on subject/object distinctions, and uncovers the assumption of subjective autonomy as a mechanism to police boundaries. What is at stake is not only the protection of one's own body from encroachments, but a denial of the leakiness between one's self and others. In either case, the instability of any foundational claims undercuts any appeal to authority made in the name of homogeneous unities, be they on the level of the individual or of the general category. Neither personal identity nor gender assignment is sufficient to ground value except in so far as it is self-consciously provisional and sensitive to change, and that alone should alert us to the violence of imposing any set of supposedly universal values.

Chapter 6

Leaks and flows
NRTs and the postmodern body

Throughout the foregoing discussion of the developments of a
specifically body-conscious feminist postmodernism, I have been
concerned to mark its implications for ethics. In particular, the
ethics of health care, which both are and are not body-centred,
have been problematised both for their abstract universalist claims
and for their inherent gender bias. Once what have been taken
by liberal humanist accounts to be secure and stable identities
and fixed subject positions are opened to a deconstructionist interrogation, then the issue of sameness and difference which has
underwritten traditional ethics loses its power. The demise both
of the unified and coherent subject, and of homogeneous categories to which such subjects might be assigned, has demanded a
reconstruction, not just of moral agency, but of the very possibility of ethical codes. What I have suggested as the basis for a
more appropriate ethic is a responsibility towards differences not
as the disembodied sites of diverse claims, but as an awareness
of the irreducible but fluid bodily investments which ground our
own provisional being in the world and our interactions with
others.

It is precisely because of the centrality of embodiment in the
feminist attention to the issue of subjectivity and selfhood, that I
shall turn now to a consideration of some aspects of the new
reproductive technologies (NRTs). However little else they have
in common, all are concerned in more or less sophisticated ways
with diversifying those limited things of which particular bodies
seem capable. In other words, they start from the point of
disrupting what is apparently given, and moreover they have
as their aim the production of new lives, and potentially new
subjectivities. The spaces and boundaries between bodies may be

radically varied by an array of present and potential interventions. Among those techniques implicated are, for example, the transplantation of ovarian and foetal tissue, the use of surrogacy which results in a separation between genetic, gestational and social motherhood, or the development of transgenic reproduction. As old distinctions, supposedly guaranteed by a fixed biology, fragment, so new but equally unstable ones arise.

What makes NRTs effectively postmodern in their own right is just that refusal to accept the notion of an unchanging natural body, and their capacity to problematise the grounds of (self) identity. Nonetheless, those same technologies have failed in general to generate any explicitly postmodernist response to their epistemological and ethical implications, with the result that existing frameworks of analysis have proved inadequate to the task. Wherever NRTs are practised, official committees of enquiry – the Warnock Committee (1984) is the best known in Great Britain – have been set up to try to resolve the myriad of unfamiliar ethical problems that have arisen by attempting to understand them within the familiar paradigms of liberal humanism. The continuing appeal to notions such as freedom, choice, property interests, equal rights and so on depends on the notion of individual, rational and transparent self-interest as the basis of agency. What is not considered, but what a feminist postmodernism would suggest, is that changes to the body cannot operate in material isolation, but must necessarily entail a reconstruction of the self. Moreover, the ability of NRTs to cut across hitherto entrenched categories of difference (fertile/infertile; young/old; lesbian/heterosexual; and potentially human/animal) underlines the instability of modernist homogeneities. As I traced out in Chapter 1, bodies have been historically subject to reconstitution, but what NRTs specifically create and work on are bodies on which recoding is a highly visible process, and one that is inherently threatening to humanist certainties.

In illustration of my contention that the new technologies throw up dilemmas irresolvable within conventional paradigms, I shall look at two specific areas of contestation as they arise within current practices. The first, and more straightforward, of the two concerns the issue of access to NRTs, where what is at stake is the capacity to vary the grounds of motherhood. The second problematic poses the question of what constitutes identity itself, and it demonstrates the extent to which postmodern technology may already be fulfilling Haraway's vision of 'permanently partial identities and contradictory standpoints' (1990: 196). Despite Haraway's own optimism, however, the feminist confrontation with postmodern science is far from being unambiguous and it replays many of the anxieties thrown up by more abstract theory. In each of the material instances I shall consider, the bodies of women are, of course, the ground of enquiry, and what emerges is that the epistemologies and ontologies founded on sameness and difference form an inadequate basis for a postmodern ethic.

REPRODUCING THE DIFFERENCE

The issues of what is sometimes called autonomous motherhood, and in relation to that of what limits should be put on access to assisted reproduction (AR), form an important part of the ethical debate, professional and lay, around reproductive medicine in general. My purpose is to look at what is involved, first and briefly from the familiar liberal humanist framework of rights and justice, but then by employing a feminist poststructuralist approach to ask how and why difference operates here to reproduce meanings and values. What makes the issues around AR particularly pertinent for feminist enquiry is that the growing sophistication and frequency of technological intervention offer ever greater possibilities of control over women's bodies. Current feminist interest in NRTs is foreshadowed, in any case, by Shulamith Firestone's ground-breaking, and now classic, text *The Dialectic of Sex*, written at the end of the 1960s. The issue for Firestone, as it had been for de Beauvoir before her, was to identify women's oppression with the way in which reproductive biology functioned to weaken their position in the social world. Her solution, far from proposing a revaluation of pregnancy and child rearing, was to turn to the liberatory potential of what were at the time highly experimental technologies: 'the biological family unit has always oppressed women and children, but now, for the first time in history, technology has created real preconditions for overthrowing these oppressive "natural" conditions, along with their cultural reinforcements' (1979: 183).

Firestone's immediate aim is to 'make possible an honest re-examination of the ancient value of motherhood' (1979: 189), and more radically to predict a return for all – women, men and children – to a 'natural polymorphous sexuality' (ibid.: 195).

Despite, however, the added proviso that women themselves must first take control of the new techniques, she offers no indication of how that might be achieved prior to women's liberation from their biology. Her programme remains Utopian, unable to address even the undifferentiated power dynamics between women and men that her radical feminism spoke to. Moreover, the rather more complex Foucauldian understanding of power, which informs my own analysis, makes Firestone's optimism seem dangerously unfounded. Given that bodies are a prime site at which power/knowledge is exercised, we must, I think, be intrinsically cautious – though not necessarily condemnatory – about whatever parameters a new, improved notion of motherhood might take. Adapting Foucault's insight about sex, we should remain aware that reproduction too is 'managed, inserted into systems of utility, regulated for the greater good of all, made to function according to an optimum' (Foucault 1979: 24). The very concept of autonomous motherhood is then deeply contradictory. My point is that the overdetermination of motherhood has been, and may continue to be, coincident with the Irigarayan view that within a hom(m)osexual economy motherhood is inadequately thought. What underlies my analysis is the belief – and this might implicitly be shared by Firestone – that only when the stifling utilitarian identification between women and motherhood is broken will women be able to enter into the relations of reproduction on terms more expressive of feminine desire.

The phrase 'autonomous motherhood', as it is used in relation to AR, is taken to describe the state of bearing a child who will intentionally be born outside of a primary heterosexual relationship and who has been conceived other than by sexual intercourse. What is clearly implied is that the potential mother has exercised her free choice in going beyond conventional behaviour in a way that is made possible only by the advent of certain technological interventions into reproduction. Accordingly, unpartnered single women and lesbians are at the centre of the debate. It should be noted, however, that by extension, any group whose 'lifestyle' fails to satisfy the normative relations of nuclear family life – namely, disabled people, sex workers, the very poor, certain minority ethnic groups and so on – may find themselves marginalised and potentially excluded from AR programmes. I shall argue that despite the putative appeal to clinical justifications for restricting access to AR, the substantive issues are socially and discursively encoded. My analysis is focused on the situation in Great Britain, though several of its features will be familiar to women in other countries.

The common understanding of the range of reproductive services classed as AR is that they are a form of medical treatment for full or partial infertility, and that this factor alone is sufficient to justify the exclusion of at least the majority of would-be autonomous mothers. Disinclination to enter into heterosexual intercourse and/or partnership is self-evidently a social and moral choice, whereas infertility is posed as a clinical condition requiring an appropriate medical response. Such an apparently simple positivist reading masks, however, several salient features which might cause us to reassess just where the limits of the eligibility of recipients lie. Clearly, the restrictions that are imposed largely to exclude non-heterosexual and non-partnered women – and this has at least become publicly acknowledged since the advent of the Human Fertilisation and Embryology Authority (HFEA) – are made on moral grounds for which there are no relevant objective correlatives. First, it must be noted that by standard definitions of infertility as the failure to conceive after one year's unprotected intercourse, as many as 15 per cent of all women of child-bearing age worldwide are deemed infertile. There is little reason to suppose that, with respect to those whose infertility is attributed to non-infectious causes, the incidence among lesbians and other excluded women differs greatly in each area from that among privileged heterosexual women.[1] Certainly, a far smaller proportion of the former may actively seek to bear children, but for those who do infertility is no less a problem. Further, for the simplest procedure of artificial insemination by either partner or donor, it is the case that apart from those women whose infertility is circumvented by the insemination of a third party – that is, by use of a surrogate – none of the women who are 'treated' is actually infertile. In other words, none is included in the 15 per-cent infertility rate mentioned above. Moreover, it has increasingly become the case that for more complex procedures such as IVF programmes, which involve substantial invasion of the woman's body, together with much decreased chance of achieving a live birth, the woman herself may nevertheless be fully fertile.[2] It is the male partners, of those women in heterosexual relationships, who are infertile or impotent. In short, the presence of female infertility does not in fact serve as a necessary criterion for inclusion in an AR programme.

The second major point is that it is not in any case, strictly speaking, the medical condition of infertility that is being treated for either women or men. The purpose of AR is not either to alleviate or cure infertility itself, but to satisfy a social desire for a child. Once that is acknowledged, then there is no reason to disqualify from treatment any woman who either does not herself fit the putative medical profile of infertility, or who has no infertile partner whose condition she is somehow supposed to share. The desire to reproduce (the so-called 'maternal instinct') is, after all, something which all women are supposed to feel, regardless of their medical or social status. It is interesting to note too that the utilitarian ethicist Peter Singer has anticipated the objection that resources should be allocated on the basis of need – minimally defined here by subfertility – by suggesting that any woman whose desire is great enough to undergo willingly what may be an extensive, intrusive and complex series of treatments should be defined as needing AR (Singer and Wells 1983: 195). And more recently another arch-utilitarian has argued more generally that 'need' should be interpreted as 'capacity to benefit' (Williams 1994). By that criterion there is again no distinction to be made between the fertile and infertile.

There are, of course, legitimate biomedical considerations regarding the ultimate success of any procedure which must arguably be taken into account, but these aside, the issue of restricted access is social rather than clinical. One protocol used by St Mary's Clinic, Manchester, for example, and cited in a subsequent court case seeking a judicial review of access criteria,[3] lists regularity of ovulation, cause of infertility, accessibility of ovaries, and the height–weight ratio of the recipient as medical criteria for selection for IVF. On the other hand, its reference to the absence of major physical or psychological illness, and to an age limit for both female and male participants are debatably relevant medical considerations; while the length of relationship, absence of prior children, residency restrictions, absence of previous attempts, and fulfilment of adoption criteria are all clearly social factors. Moreover, heterosexual coupledom is assumed throughout, with the effect that non-normative applicants are not so much excluded as made invisible within the terms of consideration.

What is clear is that the general limitation of services to partnered (sometimes even to married) heterosexual women shows that AR is intended not to benefit the individual woman, who either cannot or will not, for whatever reason, conceive through sexual intercourse, but to reinforce the patterns of normativity vested in the heterosexual nuclear family. In the majority of cases, of course, the two concerns coincide, but where women's interests do diverge from the norm, then what is held to be the public interest in reproduction within the heterosexual nuclear family has long been enforced by custom and is now enforced by law. With the exception of GIFT, which is an unexplained anomaly, all forms of AR are now governed by the Human Fertilisation and Embryology Act (1990). While Section 2 (1) of the Act lays down that services are provided for 'the purpose of assisting women to carry children', Section 13 (5) states: 'A woman shall not be provided with treatment services unless account has been taken of the welfare of any child who may be born as a result of the treatment (including the need of that child for a father).' While optimistic feminists may clutch at the straw of a legal quibble around the precise wording – 'that child' – in the final clause, it is nevertheless evident that the discourse of 'normal' family life is given wholly intentional precedence over any other considerations. Indeed, the emergence, in political and journalistic discourse, of the phrase 'pretended families', as widely applied to lesbian and gay familial arrangements, sets up not simply a preferred, but a 'true' standard.

Under the 1990 Act the assistance of advanced reproductive technologies may only be offered by licensed clinics whose continued registration and operation are governed by the HFE Authority. It is intended that guidance on the proper conduct of activities, which cover of course a whole range of technological intervention and experimentation, will be derived from the statutory code of conduct which, as Section 13 (5) indicates, privileges among other things the normative status of the heterosexual family. From the point of view of the law, donor insemination, as a low-tech procedure, is difficult to control and no attempt has been made, despite some earlier fears, to legislate against self-insemination. Nonetheless, the prudent reluctance of women to risk using fresh semen, untested for HIV, means in effect that a greatly increased proportion of those women who would previously have avoided the system altogether, are now constrained to use formal, and therefore monitored, health services. At the very same time, the pitifully small number of non-profit-making clinics – six in early 1991 at the time of the Act – which were prepared to treat lesbians, has been further reduced by the withdrawal of donor insemination (DI) services provided, and hitherto vigorously defended, by the British Pregnancy Advisory Service (BPAS). Whether that was done in anticipation of licensing difficulties, in response to the concurrent media-inspired scandal of 'virgin births',[4] or, as BPAS claims, as part of an overall review of the charity's long-term strategy, is unclear.

What is evident, however, is that the parameters of motherhood are a matter of disciplinary control. The mobilisation of AR in the service of what Foucault names bio-power (1979: 140–1) encompasses what are two seemingly contradictory moves. The power/knowledge which, on the one hand, opens up the closure of 'natural' procreation and enables some previously excluded women to situate themselves as mothers, on the other actually constructs and reinforces a limited category of 'desirable' mothers. As the conditions of reproduction are themselves varied to include more women, and in effect to bring their individual bodies under technologies of domination, so too all women are further inserted into the regulatory control of motherhood as an element of the social body. Effectively, the institution and meaning of motherhood is brought ever deeper into the realm of controlling normativities. The deployment of power is, then, both productive in constituting new effects and a corresponding set of desires, and repressive in setting up new exclusions which operate to some extent through legal prohibitions, but more importantly through the discursive control of meaning.

For the sake of simplicity – though the argument is clearly extensible – I shall take the low-tech procedure of DI as the paradigm case. What has been known as artificial insemination (AI) has been available in Great Britain as a clinical treatment for women at least since the 1930s,[5] although it was not until the 1960s when simple AI was used in conjunction with ovulation drugs that it became more widely known and used. It has been obtainable since 1968 under the NHS subject to varying degrees of restriction, although the simplicity of the technique has meant that professional monopoly of its administration has always been contested. For feminists the importance of maintaining putative control over our own bodies has encouraged the use of self-insemination, though where the wish for autonomous motherhood is concerned there may be, on that unproblematised level, paradoxically, some advantage in using formal provision. As Thomas Laqueur has pointed out, the involvement of a clinician in what is otherwise an overtly social transaction may serve to 'depaternalise' sperm (1990b: 217). He makes no comment on the well-documented tendency of male clinicians to 'father' AR conceptions, but simple insemination may lend itself less readily to such professional fantasies. In any case, although under the new law certain features of genetic identity are made available to recipients and subsequent children, donor anonymity remains protected.

It is, of course, precisely the issue of paternity, the effective absence of a male progenitor, which has become the focus of the intermittent bouts of outrage in the moral and social discourse which both represents and constructs the notion of DI. The terms of the debate disclose a deep-seated fear of autonomous motherhood as something fundamentally subversive. The Feversham Committee declared, for example, that 'knowledge that there is uncertainty about the fatherhood of some is a potential threat to the security of all' (1960: 66), while the Council for Science and Society, reporting in 1984, opined: 'AID to single women will increase the social problems of child-care and welfare, and the encouragement of lesbian families can be seen as a threat to normal family life, to say nothing of both instances failing to provide a nurturing father-figure' (1984: 61). In both cases what is to be resisted is the potential to undermine the closure of existing categories of difference. And paradoxically the anxieties produced by that conservatism may be paralleled by a feminist apprehension that the diversification of reproductive potential will result not in increased female autonomy, but in the insertion of women into new patterns of normativity.

More recently the same type of public anxiety surfaced again in Great Britain with the media exposure of the use of AR by unpartnered single women and lesbians, some of whom were labelled 'virgin mothers'. It was thought bad enough to want a child without the physical presence of a father, but clearly quite outrageous to avoid male penetration altogether. The sanctimonious tone of much of the British press has tried to link the bypassing of heterosexual relations with an inherent female neurosis or immaturity, selfishness or irresponsibility;[6] in other words, with a less than stable hold on personhood as defined in its classic Western rationalist sense. But what is at issue here is not that the subjectivity of women is undermined, for in reproduction as elsewhere the female body is subjected rather than subject, but that male hegemony is threatened. What seems to be happening is that the legitimation of that controlling power in the utilitarian sphere of maintaining 'public' (and identifiably male) interest in certain familial norms is threatened by the invasion into it of a previously distinct 'private' world of diverse individual and female sexual behaviour. It is not just, as Mary Jacobus would have it, that such responses serve to expose both '[the] gap between feminine desire and conception, and between conception and maternal desire' – which in turn disturbs the phallocratic construction of 'a unified coherent subject' (Jacobus 1990: 11); but rather that the limits of the highly constrained subjectivity tolerated in women as mothers are destabilised by the infiltration of a quasi-autonomous desire into the realm of procreation. The recognition that women might be the subjects of desire, rather than simply objects constructed by the desire of others, is itself an important marker for female moral agency; but where the masculine economy of reproduction is clearly vulnerable to a deconstructionist challenge is when that female desire refuses to be contained within the bounds of the other. Autonomous motherhood both decisively rejects normative biological reproduction, and situates a desire which threatens to leak out into the very centre of the phallocratic order.

As part of its privileging of the heterosexual family as the site of reproduction, the dominant discourse does nevertheless have a place for one signifier of female desire. It is expressed as the highly bounded notion of maternal instinct, that supposedly universal experience of women which, like heterosexuality itself, is endowed with the attribute of being an objective natural reality. If female desire is to be acknowledged at all, then its teleological limitation is to the socially efficacious realm of maternity, and to men; yet even those apparently distinct sites may be merged in the phallocratic imagination. Freud's conflation of babies and penises, as objects of desire, expresses perfectly the male strategy of bringing women's sexuality under control. Commenting on Freud's article 'Femininity' in *New Lectures on Psycho-analysis*, Luce Irigaray remarks: 'The child ... appears merely to be a *penis-product and penis-substitute*. The contribution of woman's germ cells, the part played by her sex organs, her body, in the formation of the child, are ... totally ignored' (1985a: 74). And psychoanalysis is just one among the elaborate and multiple discourses of medicine, the law, religion and biology which work together to hold in place a power/knowledge regime that operates to ensure male control over female bodies. The problem, of course, arises in the conceptual conflict between the notion that all women naturally want babies and the public denial of the validity, morally and socially, of certain forms of motherhood, including autonomous motherhood. Where the area of fertility services is concerned the state's response is to restrict access to those deemed suitable mothers, which effectively means those women who express their 'instincts' in the proper form.[7]

The justification for such restrictions clearly cannot rest on clinical grounds, so appeal is made to a linked series of moral arguments. The first resort is to the validity of society's interest in the 'normal' family which takes the form of a straightforward appeal to public morality, which is in any case privileged in liberal democracies. The Warnock Report (1984), for example, which formed the ideological basis of the subsequent Human Fertilisation and Embryology Act, seems to support the position that any action which can be conceived as shocking or offensive to public opinion must count as harmful even when it involves no intrinsic harm. Mary Warnock herself, writing elsewhere, defends her stance in the report in just such terms, and adds a comment which makes clear the problematic of plural differences: 'the centre of anxiety for most people ... is whether we actually like the idea of a society within which all these different kinds of families are acceptable' (1985: 149). Second, appeal is made to the question-begging legal policy adopted by both US and British courts of giving precedence to the child's best interests. The final appeal is to scarce resources, which though plausibly a real consideration in high-tech interventions, can scarcely operate on the DI level. In any case, the argument relies on a predetermined definition of need which is supposed to disqualify from consideration all 'autonomous mothers' – that is, those assumed to be fertile, and therefore capable of reproducing by conventional means. But not only does that argument offer an oversimplistic identification of a category of 'fertile' women, it also fails to justify its own utilitarian basis. If the moral parameters are to be set by the maximisation of benefit, as utilitarianism demands, then there is no reason here to suppose that autonomous mothers would benefit less from AR procedures. And as noted already, Peter Singer (Singer and Wells 1983), himself a committed utilitarian, has effectively repositioned the satisfaction of desire – rather than need – as the operative utility. Nonetheless, fertility services are restricted, in fact, on a basis that unremittingly marginalises certain lifestyles, like that of sex workers, or sexual identities, such as lesbian. Plainly eligibility for motherhood is intended to coincide with normative standards of sexual practice. In other words, the sexual behaviour of the woman becomes the template for good and bad motherhood.

Now the standard way to challenge this 'lifestyle' restriction would be through the liberal humanist notion of a morality centred on the autonomous individual as the holder of specified rights. The following considerations might ensue:

1 The state and medical profession have no right to interfere with the freedom of the individual except to prevent significant harm.[8] What empirical research there is – see, for example, Golombok and Rust (1986) in the United Kingdom, and McGuire and Alexander (1985) in the United States – shows that children born into single or lesbian couple homes show no disturbance of psycho-sexual identity or behaviour. Committed feminists might well find this concordance with the conventional and restricted developmental stereotypes depressing, but more to the point, there is here no evidence that either the child's or the state's interest in stability is harmed. Indeed, it is instructive to note that the state's interest has occasionally been positively served by encouraging unrestricted AR. In the years of the Second World War, for example, a pro-natalist MP, speaking in the House of Commons, recommended AID for women 'who would like to have children without marrying and without sinning' (reported in 'Medical notes in Parliament', *British Medical Journal*, August 1943: 219). In short, the 'harm' approach offers no consistent justification for countermanding the choices of the mother as an independent moral agent.

2 If the notional right to reproduce exists for any woman, then it may, by extension, be claimed by all women.[9]

3 A more familiar formulation for feminists might be the long-contested claim for the right to bodily self-determination.

The immediate drawback with the last two points is that given the conceptual difficulty of grounding a naturally occurring right

– which must presuppose both some essentialist character and an appeal to transcendental authority – liberal opponents of restrictive clauses are in effect relying on contract or custom rights. In other words, the difficulty for those women seeking a more open approach to access criteria is that rights, almost by definition, conform to a given order of things. And as Gena Corea puts it: 'any discussion of "rights" . . . assumes a society in which there are no serious differences of power and authority between individuals' (1988: 3). Far from the equality supposedly guaranteed to the holders of rights, there is at very least a hierarchy in which, as Carol Smart puts it in her analysis of the parallel context of child custody disputes, 'rights to *specific* forms of family life are justified while certain individual rights of choice and autonomy are redefined as destructive of the very right to family life' (1989: 23; my emphasis). Hitherto marginalised groups can claim putative identification with the standard of good motherhood, as already supposedly exemplified by married heterosexual women, and equal rights as women, only on the following conditions: first, they must neither change nor challenge the inherent standards of value; and second, they must deny the specificity of their own position. In other words, rights are only available to those who are encompassed within the economy of the same.

The next recourse offered within liberal humanism is an appeal to justice, but that too does nothing to contest the referent standard, relying instead on some notion of abstract equality. The concept of justice may operate, of course, according to a variety of criteria, such as rights, need, desert and so on. What makes it superficially attractive to feminists with reference to NRTs is that even when the operation of selection protocols is identified as establishing treatment not as a right or need, but as a privilege (Overall 1987: 170), it would be unjust to deny a priori that privilege to certain groups. And further it can claim that it is unjust to impose discriminatory conditions on those who conceive by means of AR as opposed to those doing so by sexual intercourse. The claim is that everyone is to be treated equally unless individually disabling factors emerge. Corea's point about differential power is no less relevant here, and is particularly pertinent in a society in which the greater part of AR treatment is offered only by commercial clinics at sometimes prohibitive cost. But what is most important is not that some conceptions of justice may fail to challenge the discriminatory provisions of the free market, but that the *prima facie* assumption of equality fails to ask 'equal to what?'. It relies, once again, on privatising individual sexuality, and on suppressing the differences between women.

From the modernist perspective, the situation, then, is that restriction of access is *justified* in terms of marginalised groups being different from morally normative groups; and *contested* on the basis that really, as far as it matters, everyone is the same. In short, the organising principles are the ones of sameness and difference, just those which a deconstructionist will wish to interrogate. The initial stages of a poststructuralist critique assert the following:

1 that the reliance on abstract ahistorical principles of moral behaviour is misconstrued, and should be superseded by an understanding of such principles as specific and discursively constructed;
2 that there is no underlying real nature of things: meaning is constructed only in language;
3 that all arguments predicated on binary oppositions, such as natural/unnatural, heterosexual/homosexual, good mother/ bad mother, conceal a hierarchy in which one term is consistently privileged over the other. Thus heterosexual, married, monogamous as the accepted referent standard for reproduction does not simply claim its own centrality but is taken as the guarantor of good motherhood. And the discursive marginalisation of its others – lesbian, single and so on – lays the foundation for material discrimination against autonomous motherhood. And it is no surprise to find that what is consistently marginalised is any position which does not fit the gender norms essential to patriarchy.

The familiar modernist use of the concept of difference presupposes two things that underwrite its justificatory claim to be neutral and objective: on the one hand, the claim that language expresses some prior reality; and on the other that difference itself can be universalised, that something really is either *A* or *not-A*. As I outlined in Chapter 3, poststructuralism denies both these claims and asserts instead two quite different points. First, even if there is a 'real' world, we can make sense of it only through language. There is then no unmediated access to facts, and we cannot speak of natural conditions or essence, but only of the symbolic constructs of language. Accordingly 'reproduction', 'maternal instinct' and 'motherhood' are never neutral, unmediated concepts but always already compromised by the inherent concerns of phallogocentric discourse. Second, where the notion of universal differences relies both on a closure of meaning and on clearly defined boundaries between terms, Derrida has shown that neither complete separation nor totalisation is possible. The idea of definition in the sense of both epistemic content and fixed limits is destabilised by the trace of the other, so that meaning is at best provisional, and boundaries fluid. There can be, then, no rigid universalist divisions, either of value – good/bad – or of material categories. Moreover, in the unstable economy of *différance* the suppressed margins continually encroach on the centre.

So what could this mean for a feminist ethics of reproduction? The appropriate deconstructionist manoeuvre is to insist that difference *simpliciter*, as an expression of supposedly universal categories, is an untenable construct which must be replaced by a plural notion of differences. On a poststructuralist reading we may accept that lesbians, for example, are different from heterosexual women in some consistent though never fixed nor essentialist senses, but not that they are different as a universal category. Rather, the differences describe multiple diversities. And further, it is not simply the differences between groups which are plural and fluid, but that neither term – lesbian nor heterosexual – speaks to an homogeneous group. Moreover, if what conventionally counts as good or right is determined by its association with the familiar male-constructed standards of liberal humanism which privilege the self-contained unitary one over against excess, then as Luce Irigaray has demonstrated, female sexuality, in its expression of female desire, has always threatened to break those bounds (Irigaray 1985b: 29–30). To the male world of order, autonomous motherhood, like lesbianism itself, just is excessive. Thus, however we are encoded in phallogocentric discourse, both the categorical distinctions drawn between women, and the homogeneity of those categories, are frustrated by both differences and *différance*. It can make no sense, therefore, to apply universal a priori judgments like good and bad mother.

In terms of applied ethics, what I am suggesting is that the deconstruction of difference between groups might lead to moral considerations based not on the false security of universals but on a recognition of diversity among women, and of the singularity of each woman. It would mean that marginalised women should no longer need to deny their difference in the tentative hope of being accepted as the same; but nor should they claim a common counter-identity. The issue is one of individual specificity, both for themselves and indeed for the partnered heterosexual women who occupy the centre. It is not that I wish to reinstate the sovereign individual so crucial to liberal humanism, but to insist that identity itself is discursively constructed, never fixed but always in process. Nonetheless, as a feminist project, the deconstruction of the monolithic differences of language is perhaps unlikely to affect policy directly. What it can do, however, is to open up a discursive space in which to pluralise the notion of motherhood and challenge both the 'grand narratives' of normative heterosexuality, and ultimately the material consequences of that hegemony. Provisionally, at least, we can seek to outline the multiple discourses of needs/desires as the basis for working towards a proper regard for specificity. And provisionally the operation of access conditions to AR resources which took such diversity into account would indeed be a more just one.

My use of the qualifier 'provisionally' is made here advisedly, for what has just been outlined is surely no more than the second stage of deconstruction which I identified earlier as a necessary but insufficient step. That is why we should still feel uncomfortable with Sara Ruddick's optimistic assertion that 'a more open and efficient use of artificial insemination, combined with more flexible sexual mores and an insistent gay politics, allow women increasing control over the role of men in procreation and mothering' (Ruddick 1990b: 222). It is my contention that the feminist agenda must go further than the appropriation of culture for our own ends; it must deconstruct the implicit link between women and nature by challenging the appeal to biological determinism which shows itself in the notion of maternal instinct. The danger is that as technological intervention increasingly enables almost any woman to achieve pregnancy, fertility itself would become prescriptive. As Marilyn Strathern puts it: 'To imagine an absence of desire would be an affront to the means that exist to satisfy it' (1992: 37). In other words, the 'failure to establish a rationale for childlessness' (Stanworth 1990: 297) leaves women still subject to a hegemonic discourse regardless of who controls the means to motherhood. It is only when the notion of natural instincts, of given essence, is subjected to deconstruction, that the multiple determinations of the desire to reproduce – or not – may be addressed.

What is needed is the displacement of the whole cultural code that implicitly identifies women only as mothers, and sets there the limited ground for female subject positions and female agency. As I indicated at the beginning of this section, the simple diversification of the relations of reproduction, which might result from contesting restrictive access conditions, may simply invite the net of regulatory power to spread wider. We must, I think, regard the celebration of unproblematised autonomous motherhood with some scepticism. To break the closure and unity of acceptable motherhood is an important step, but the further aim must surely be to disturb the repressive identity between women and motherhood as it is understood in the male social order. It is not simply the ground, but the terms of moral debate that must be reassessed. An ethic of *différance* demands no less.

What is at a stake in a postmodernist feminism involves always an element of risk, for what must be given up in favour of the incalculable are not just the repressive aspects of women's lives, but also the very things that may bring meaning and certainty. For all of us there is a sense in which our own bodies and our own personal identities may be the only things of which we feel sure, that do seem in a common-sense way to be outside the text. Though low-tech NRTs at the level of intervention discussed above may signal a move towards differences, those differences remain assimilable within all but the most conservative models of feminism. The recognition of the diversity of women is now a common aspect of feminist theory. Nonetheless, as I have signalled, more disruptive implications are never far behind, and these are more clearly evident in my second area of enquiry. The dilemmas I shall go on to address position identity and subjectivity at the forefront of concern and mark them as that which distinguishes postmodernist feminism from other approaches. What is at issue, indeed what is risked, is the ability to know oneself as a subject at all.

MIS(SED)CONCEPTIONS: NRTS AND ONTOLOGICAL ANXIETY.

In Foucauldian analytics, as I have shown in Chapter 1, sexuality stands both as the privileged site in the formation of subjectivity, and as the primary focus of the power/knowledge regime. If, as I now propose, this notion can be extended to the specificities of the reproductive body, then the (temporal/spatial) intervention of the new reproductive technologies, which range from simple insemination to genetic engineering, must inevitably problematise the existing nexus. It is not, of course, that I want to draw any naïve distinction between the 'natural' and the 'technological' but rather to look at the way in which some recent developments in this specific area of biomedicine take their place in the field of forces that constitute the construction/(re)production of identity. Feminist responses to NRTs are by no means uniform, or even predictable from their particular theoretical bases, and concern about the place of technological intervention may not explicitly ask questions of ontology. Nevertheless, I discern an underlying reference to what it is to be a subject in a woman's body, and the issue I will address is whether or not ontological anxiety is the appropriate feminist response to NRTs, and what that might tell us about an ethics of the embodied self.

That the operation of NRTs does raise important ethical issues at every level is uncontested by all but the most unreclaimed of practitioners, but what will concern me here is premised on the consideration that an ethics for the postmodern age can no longer be conflated with traditional morality. Rather, my concern is with an ethics of the particular self in resistance to totalising and universalising discourses and practices (Braidotti 1991a). I do not understand that resistance as, and perhaps it cannot be, a personally liberatory endeavour, but rather one which continually seeks to uncover the constitutive mechanisms of truth and knowledge as they construct and position the individual within social and scientific fields. What is at issue is the ground on which traditional notions of right and wrong, good and evil are put into play, rather than any attempt to problematise the attribution of such terms. And in so far as medical practice entails ways of thinking and knowing that legitimise 'the development of procedures of normalisation upon the living bodies of actual human beings' (Rawlinson 1987: 391), my approach, as before, draws strongly on the work of Foucault, albeit with a necessary caution. What is absent from his analysis is a proper consideration of two further points of crucial importance to any feminist deconstruction of health-care practices. First, insufficient attention is paid to questions of difference. Though Foucault critiques the universalisation of operative standards, he falls short of adequately theorising either plural differences or, more importantly, sexual difference, particularly as it might express the radically other rather than the mirror of the selfsame. His analysis demands recognition for the multiplicity of the experiencing body, but fails to situate difference at the ethical core. From this emerges my second and repeated point of contention, that Foucault, despite his discursive concentration on the disciplinary practices focused on the female body, is nevertheless gender-indifferent in his approach. What he consistently fails to acknowledge is that the (re)productive bodies at the centre of his analysis – in *The History of Sexuality*, volume 1, for example – are women's bodies, and that the power/knowledge regime grounded there is contextualised by the differential power relations between women and men. The effacement of difference in this sense reflects the operations of phallocentric knowledge and represents an unreconstructed obstacle to our understanding. Luce Irigaray writes:

> [the] domination of the philosophic logos stems in large part from its power to *reduce all others to the economy of the Same* ... from its power to *eradicate the difference between the sexes* in systems that are self-representative of a 'masculine subject'.
>
> (1985b: 74)

And precisely the same could be said of scientific practice. What I have been suggesting, then, in line with Irigaray and contrary to Foucault, is that the recovery of sexual difference is crucial to a feminist ethic.

But let us return to the question of ontological anxiety, by which I mean the apprehension that one's very sense of self-identity might be under threat. Before proceeding, a few observations on the parameters of identity are necessary. I offer no definitive exposition, but simply mark that my use of the term ranges from its Latin root *idem*, meaning the same – in other words, everything that is not other – through to a partial and strategic elision with the term 'subjectivity'; that is, with the self-experiencing self, and its further implications of knowing, speaking and acting. And though the boundaries of the individual body may not exhaust the possibilities of self-identity, that body is nevertheless taken as the central focus, particularly for women to whom transcendence is most often denied. I take it as axiomatic that identity is always gendered, but shall propose that it is in large part an unreconstructed and unwitting collusion with the male discourse of *oppositional* identity that has lead one major and possibly the dominant feminist response – as represented most vocally world-wide by the group FINRRAGE[10] – to view NRTs with foreboding. It is not my intention to suggest that FINRRAGE has got it all wrong, and indeed the exposure of the often obscured dangers and liabilities of NRTs is of enormous ethical consequence in the traditional sense. Rather, my concern is to critique the basis of their analysis in that it assumes certain fixed modes of female being. In adopting a postmodernist perspective – though always aware of the efficacy of strategic alternatives – I shall argue that the view that implicitly counterposes natural with technological reproduction, as FINRRAGE does, relies on a closure of identity that in fact may inhibit women's interests. Moreover, that type of humanist focus obscures that what really constitutes the moral issue, the reason why NRTs can be so unsettling, is an ethics of difference.

Before looking at what is at stake for identity in its relation to reproduction, I want to reiterate that I take the latter to be both a thoroughly discursive construction, and the material site of embodied experience. There is, in other words, no given 'natural' state of reproduction, but nor is it simply a set of free-floating signifiers. Indeed, the temptation to dichotomise the real and ideal simply mirrors the view that Irigaray has identified as founda-tional to male hegemony: 'the mother-matter gives birth only to images, the Father-Good only to the real' (1985a: 301). Certainly reality always eludes us, is always deferred, but that is not to say that our constructions are not embedded in solid material prac-tices. The specificity of the female body is central to any understanding of the meaning of reproduction as the locus of identity, but that does not mean that the issues, ontological or ethical, can be unproblematically resolved by reference to biolog-ical underpinnings.

In any case what soon becomes apparent is that in the partial reconceptualisation, promoted by masculinist science and the popular media, of reproduction as a technological rather than natural process, the individual female body is seen as increasingly irrelevant (Kirejczyk and van der Ploeg 1992). It is not simply the maternal, but also paternal and foetal, identity which is at stake, for while the first may be under threat, the latter are promoted. One clear indication, that I have already mentioned, of the growing emphasis given to the reproduction of paternal identity is the by now widespread use of IVF as the first-choice option in the 'treatment' of subfertile and infertile men (Lorber 1989). In this paradigm of maternal effacement, the 'treated' (woman's) body is not of course coincident with the infertile body, and will indeed be in most cases clinically normal. In other words, a medical problem emanating in the male body – in that low sperm count, poor motility, or misshapen sperm may inhibit unassisted fertilisation – is 'solved' by intervention into the female body. And where in the past donor insemination, with its inherent problematisation of paternity, was the standard intervention, now IVF, a far more expensive, intrusive and potentially dangerous procedure, with a much reduced probability of resulting in live birth, is the socially preferred option.[11] The literature around NRTs, aimed at both practitioners and prospective clients, explicitly justifies and normalises the process as preserving paternal identity.[12] At the same time, the woman, as the proximate patient of NRTs, is scarcely acknowledged as having any subject identity at all. At best, as Kirejczyk puts it: 'The pregnancy, until now so intimately related to the feminine identity, becomes an attribute of a heterosexual couple' (1992: n.p.).

Now clearly this stress on coupledom partly mirrors patriarchal society's continued reluctance to acknowledge the potential of autonomous motherhood, but it speaks also to a more fundamental male desire to use women's bodies in the reproduction of their own identities. Irigaray, for example, claims: 'The use, consumption and circulation of [women's] sexualized bodies underwrite the organization and the reproduction of the social order, in which they have never taken part as "subjects"' (1985b: 84), and again that '[p]roperty, ownership, and self-definition are the attributes of the father's production' (1985a: 300). What is at work in NRTs then is the intensification of existing material and psychological pressures on maternal identity.

A yet more insidious consequence of the new technologies, as I noted in Chapter 1, is the reconstructed emphasis now given to the foetus, not just as a passive object of moral concern, but as a quasi-autonomous self. Many feminist commentators opposed to NRTs explain this as occurring within a political climate that privileges the foetus, and a market economy reliant on intervention into the reproductive process (Raymond 1987, 1990; Spallone 1989). Their case is strong; but nonetheless a yet more anxiety-provoking move seems to be at stake. As the 1984 anti-abortion video, *The Silent Scream*, illustrates, it is not just that the developing foetus is characterised as having an identity counterposed to that of the mother, but that the mother as a subject identity in her own right may be entirely absent. Moreover, that 'loss' of maternal presence is intensified as increasingly sophisticated techniques of imaging extend identity back to become an attribute of the embryo from the moment of conception (Petchesky 1987; Martin 1991). And further, though we may see the homunculi of seventeenth- and eighteenth-century gynae-cological textbooks as an historical curiosity, modern works – both scientific and popular – endow not just the gametes, but genetic material itself with sex-specific attributes of agency (Biology and Gender Study Group 1988). Yet what modern bioscience and genetics present as biology stripped bare – scanning electron microscopy, the photographic imaging of the moment of conception, the on-screen display of ultrasound and the latest developments in endoscopy – are all representations generated by the body as text. Nonetheless, where the gaze is privileged, as it arguably is in medical discourse in particular, the authority of the visual image, as an apparently direct copy of reality, greatly enhances our ability to identify the foetus as self-present. And in emphasising the disconnectedness of the gestating foetus/embryo, the effect of such imaging, I would suggest, is to *empty out* the maternal body. As Rosi Braidotti recognises, it is a paradigm case of insecure boundaries: 'Offering everything for display or show, representing the unrepresentable (like the origins of life), means producing images that displace the boundaries of space (inside/outside the mother's body) and of time (before/after birth)' (1991b: 366).

In a parallel move the framework in which pregnancy is located for medico-legal purposes increasingly privileges the foetus at the expense of the mother. In the United Kingdom, the Human Fertilisation and Embryology Act (1990) uncritically assumes that the foetus is an independent entity, worthy not just of consider-ation, but capable of bearing rights. Further, state intervention, aimed at forcing women to optimise the conditions of their preg-nancies, is implicitly predicated on the notion of foetal subjecthood. For some years the involvement of the law in many states in North America has gone beyond the UK procedure of placing projective care orders on late foetuses and has sanctioned in addition a stringent range of penalties and enforced 'treatments' against pregnant women: drug/alcohol abusers can be prosecuted for foetal abuse, for example, or forced onto rehabilitation programmes (de Wit and Corea 1990: 51; Birenbaum-Cameli 1995). The bald either/or approach – that is, the conventional difference approach – to any supposed conflict between maternal and foetal interests can lead directly to the negation of the mother's choice and agency whenever the foetus is privileged. Courts in both the United States and Great Britain have intervened to order women, regardless of lack of consent, to undergo Caesarean sections when that is medically indicated for the well-being of the prospective neonate (Rogers 1989; Callahan and Knight 1992; Draper 1993). The British case, *Re S* Family Division, 12 October 1992, in which the mother withheld consent on religious grounds but was overruled, was the first to establish that the foetus may have an independent *legal* existence before birth in addition to its existing moral claims. Although, then, the nexus of legal, religious and ethical discourse around abortion and birth has long been expressive of the conflict between two rights-bearing individuals, what is new about more recent disciplinary techniques is that the mother is increasingly effaced altogether. It is no longer a simple clash of interests, but the prioritisation of what is best for the foetus (now the unborn child) in its development in a non-specific and disembodied space. That that space is in fact the mother's womb, and that the foetus is dependent upon it and her is erased.

The expanded opportunities for body management offered by NRTs in the pursuit of both the social utilities of bio-power and the control of women are alarming in their widespread and increasingly manipulative procedures. What is particularly disturbing about many such practices, however, is the way in which they so clearly exemplify what Foucault calls 'technologies of the self'. Fuelled by the creation of new desires, these self-disciplinary techniques

permit individuals to effect, by their own means, a certain number of operations on their bodies, their own souls, their own thoughts, their own conduct, and this in a manner so as to transform themselves, modify themselves, and to attain a state of perfection, happiness, purity and supernatural power.
(Foucault 1985a: 367)

Where issues of fertility are concerned, the cultural stigmatisation of the infertile body as an object of pity or exclusion is answered by the woman's self-objectification in the context of ever more complex and sophisticated reproductive technologies. The identity of 'mother', overdetermined by a relentless cycle of fetishisation and desire, both becomes the focus of an unremitting struggle, and at the same time evades capture. Infertility is simultaneously exposed and concealed.

If one believes, as many feminists do, that the woman as gestating mother is a subject position of peculiar potency, then one must view with alarm any threat to that unique and powerful identity. What the range of NRTs does is both to demand that the normativity of the established relations of conception and gestation should be re-examined, and to threaten a radical overturning of the very concept of *in vivo* reproduction. But just as the so-called sexual revolution of the 1960s, which effectively made sex without babies a real option for women, was both liberatory and disciplinary, productive and repressive in the Foucauldian sense, so current technological developments which offer babies without sex are equally ambivalent. It would be misleading, however, to see that ambivalence as operating in either a unidirectional or homogeneous way. It is not my purpose to explore detail here, but it is difficult to believe that all the new technologies exploit women in the same way or all of the time. Moreover, in terms of the symbiotic relationship between NRTs and the power/knowledge regime, the potential advantages for women may be both material and discursive.

The *objections* to the interwoven ideology and practices of NRTs range over seeing them as:

- physically dangerous to women in terms of the use of procedures like superovulation which risk both multiple conception and ectopic pregnancy if 'successful', and increased incidence of ovarian cysts, tumours and premature menopause whether pregnancy occurs or not;
- mentally distressing due to intrusive procedures combined in most cases with an extremely low live birth rate – no more than 15 per cent for IVF, for example;
- effectively racist, classist and heterosexist in the setting up of unethical research programmes or in the discriminatory restriction of access;

- concentrating reproductive power in the hands of the male establishment;
- threatening to women's very identity.[13]

In drawing attention to the current unacceptibility of such outcomes the critique offered by FINRRAGE is crucial, but its overall agenda is directed towards a blanket rejection rather than recuperation of the NRTs. Despite a fine grasp on clinical detail, the unwillingness to make distinctions of value between the various techniques makes it clear that FINRRAGE believes them to be a threat to women *per se*. Now it seems to me that if a provisional separation of these different types of objections were possible, then in theory the grounds for most could be empirically modified, both in particular and in general, to offer a more ethically and politically acceptable model. Birke *et al.*, for example, have attempted just such a move when they suggest ways of transforming the practice of NRTs to make them more liberatory and productive, and to give women more control (1990: chapter 8 and 'Conclusions'). What would remain as the sticking point, however, is the final objection about the perceived threat to women's maternal identity. Yet even in this, a curious contradiction exists in that the FINRRAGE group, and indeed Birke *et al.*, do not acknowledge that medical discourse in general – like every technology of power – is always already constitutive of personal identity. They see NRTs therefore as *different in kind* in supposedly making an assault on what is taken to be not just a pre-given body, but also a stable subjectivity. What is masked in this construction is the transactive textuality of identity, the way in which it is constructed by, and operates through, both discursive and material forces. The separation, then, of objections into discrete categories may be strategically useful in clarifying thought, but the call neither for feminist resistance to, nor control of, NRTs will realise what is in effect an illusory identity. The issue of ontological anxiety is irreducible, and it demands a very different analysis and response.

Clearly, the concept of fertilisation, and potentially of gestation, as being somehow independent of the maternal body does speak to a radical reformulation of the discourse of reproduction, but I am by no means convinced that this represents a paradigm shift in the meanings of motherhood. There seem instead to be two possible ways of looking at it: either women have hitherto been the unique source and origin of life, and therein lies the core of our identities and our power; or that very identification of women as mothers is the proximate reason for the quasi-essentialist and historically damaging split between female-nature and male-culture. Despite a theoretical capacity to encompass either perspective, essentialist or constructivist, radical feminism is most often taken to support the former and to generate a politics based on immutable referents. Jana Sawicki, for example, often seems to make such an assumption in her oversimplified elision of the FINRRAGE analysis and radical feminist theory (Sawicki 1991: chapter 4).[14] It is worth remembering, however, that Firestone's consideration of reproductive technologies in *The Dialectic of Sex* (1979), in which she welcomes them as liberatory in their potential to free women from the embodied specificity of reproduction, is explicitly radical feminist in its perspective. That her optimistic expectations may look naïve in the light of subsequent developments, and moreover seem to concur with a masculinist view of the body, does not undermine her anticipation of the transgressive power of NRTs.

Nonetheless, the political impulse to reject NRTs wholesale surely reflects just that type of essentialist analysis which Sawicki assumes of radical feminism, for what is taken to be unacceptable about a range of such technologies is that they fundamentally disrupt the natural and proper link between the woman and her maternal identity. It is as though the patriarchy had found in NRTs the ultimate target for the erasure of women as speaking/knowing subjects, and that visualisation of the processes of fertilisation and gestation, that the evermore intimate opening up of the enclosed space of the maternal body, were enough to make women finally invisible. And it is true, the biomedical literature of NRTs is full of the imagery of male progenitors – technodocs, donors, even spermatozoa – as unified, self-present agents controlling fertilisation, achieving pregnancies and claiming birth. This usurpation of the apparent maternal function and the substitution of male agency as foundational is paralleled by the fragmentation of the maternal body under the biotechnical gaze, or even its complete absence in *in vitro* conception. Having no place, female self is dispersed, while male and foetal identity assume the positions of seer and seen.

And yet, though the technologies themselves are new, the erasure of the woman from stories of origin is, as I have indicated before, a fundamental feature of the Western logos. Irigaray writes at length of the '[e]clipse of the mother, of the place (of) becoming, whose non-representation or even disavowal upholds the absolute being attributed to the father' (1985a, 'Plato's *Hystera*': 307). What can never be acknowledged is the plenitude of the mother, the disruptive excess which threatens constantly to undermine male unity and self-presence. Even in the light of her recent allusions to a placental economy (1993b, 'On the maternal order': 38–44) and despite her long-term, arguably strategic, alignment with essentialist conceptions of the body, Irigaray need not, I think, see the technologies of reproduction as inherently counterposed to female interests. Rather they present a further challenge to *male* identity, which is precisely why there is so much at stake in their control. '*So now man struggles to be science, machine, woman, . . . to prevent any of these escaping his service and ceasing to be interchangeable*' (1985a: 232; ellipsis in original).

Irigaray is engaged fundamentally with the fluidity of boundaries, and because of her strategic concerns there is a way in which her work forms a bridge between a wholly essentialist account and the quite different problematic yielded by the alternative readings, which I offer now, of the meaning of reproduction. The simplest starts from the premise that there is nothing natural about the concept of reproduction, but that all meanings are always/already embedded in a discursive field. Nonetheless, Western humanism, as it has impinged on medical theory at least, takes as its central organising feature the belief in a stable, unified subject, which is sustained by a series of now familiar gendered and hierarchical dichotomies. Earlier waves of feminism, in facing up to those polarities, either resorted to the notion of a redistribution of power through a reversal of priorities, or contested the fixity of the categories by emphasising the constructed nature of *gender*. Although anatomical sex was seen as basic and natural – and pregnancy therefore an immutable and ahistorical characteristic of most women's lives – at least the organisation of reproduction and motherhood was open to reconstruction. The essentialist idea that women should be restricted by their biology to the dominant identity of mother, that their desire should be characterised as directed toward a single end, was recognised as a damaging limitation to the subjectivity of all women, and the basis on which women have been excluded from social and political power.

In consequence, one might expect that such an analysis should lead to a cautious welcome for NRTs in so far as they reconstruct reproduction and implicitly challenge the grounds of women's supposedly limited identity. But though the conventional relations between women and reproduction are broken down by the blurring of the distinctions between fertile and infertile, the use of surrogacy, the possibility of delayed gestation offered by embryo freezing, the potential transplantation of foetal ovarian tissue and so on, there is reason to think that far from pluralising women's identity and desire, the new technologies merely pluralise the *conditions* for motherhood. This may be no bad thing when it allows lesbian women, for example, to conceive without heterosexual intercourse, but it seems also to reinforce a single identity for all women. Against the undoubted benefit to individuals previously unable to satisfy their desire for children who are genetically linked either to themselves or to their partners, the danger is that whole new categories of women are being brought within normative parameters. As motherhood becomes a real option regardless of fertility status, age or sexuality, local heterogeneities may flourish, but overall difference disappears. And on that ground alone, NRTs would deeply offend against any postmodern feminist ethic.

In taking the analysis further along a deconstructionist path, however, two further considerations emerge. The first, which I have been stressing from the beginning, is that biology itself is not somehow outside discourse, which is not to say that nothing 'real' happens, but that reality is always deferred, always mediated, always constructed. As such the elision of woman-mother is an effect of phallocentric discourse, seemingly universalised across the bodies of all women, but always having local and specific application. Second, the hierarchical polarities function not merely to sustain the power of the male humanist subject, but also to create him. Given that all boundaries depend on exclusion, and in so far as male identity is predicated on mind rather than body, the mother-matter, mother-other is the necessary condition of the self-same. But as poststructuralist theory has demonstrated, those boundaries are inherently unstable, and simple difference gives way to *différance*. The subject – both male and female – is always non-identical with itself, so that the issue of identity is already and necessarily problematised. What NRTs may do in material terms is to make manifest both the discursive leakage between categories and the lack of definition at the heart of each individual. Moreover, as Donna Haraway has pointed out, women have always had 'trouble counting as individuals in modern western discourses. Their personal, bounded individuality is compromised by their bodies' troubling talent for making other bodies, whose individuality can take precedence over their own' (1989: 39). So although NRTs may intensify that undecidability, female bodies always already frustrate the desire for identity. The other within the same is a necessary feature of all endogenous reproduction, breaking boundaries, disrupting identity, postmodern all along.

The question to ask, then, is not whether we should oppose NRTs for the sake of our selves – for in reproduction the female body has always been more subjected than subject – nor even whether we would be better off freed from the putative biological strait-jacket, but why we should attach ontological anxiety to reproduction at all. Although, as Kaplan puts it, '[t]he de-essentializing of subjectivity and, in a related move, of identity, should free women ... of their simultaneous subordination and fetishization' (1992: 219), the issue of identity has strategic rather than ontological importance. The signifier 'mother' is already indeterminate; and if there is in any case no one site of identity, then we must relocate ourselves in multiple and dispersed subject positions. To focus the sense of self around one single issue, to insist on and defend the unity and closure of the maternal subject, can only collude with the phallocratic insistence on identity as that which excludes the other. But women, as Irigaray has argued, just are excessive to all forms of male discourse, and the multiple determinants of female desire and female identity cannot be encompassed in any single location: 'the geography of her pleasure is far more diversified, more multiple in its differences, more complex, more subtle, than is commonly imagined – in an imaginary rather too narrowly focused on sameness' (Irigaray 1985b: 28). As Irigaray suggests, the move away from the focus of maternity does not mean that our sexed bodies are of no importance. Moreover, if the political and social asymmetry between women and men is predicated on particular representations of the female body, then our resistance must start at the same point. Where the feminist project is one of recuperating difference as irreducible, multiple and non-hierarchical, we must insist that the female subject is neither disembodied nor desexualised.

The attempt to draw distinctions between the materiality of women's lives and the ontological project is in the end futile. And it is now clearer why the possibility, that I gestured towards earlier, of making a separation between the various feminist objections to NRTs will not hold. So given that NRTs do indeed appear to threaten the physical and socio-political well-being of women – though it must always be acknowledged that individual women may experience them in wholly positive terms – should we, as feminists, oppose their development? Not necessarily, for just as issues of identity are already highly contested in both the symbolic and material sense, so the disciplinary techniques of NRTs as practised on the bodies of women cannot be construed as univalent. As Foucault has made clear, any new procedure in the power/knowledge regime of any discourse, be it medical, legal or political, generates its own sites of resistance.[15] Nothing is simply repressive nor wholly encompassed in the service of the dominant, but is always provisional, unstable and epistemologically plural. The micro-practices of bio-power, where 'sex' (for which we may read 'reproduction') 'is located at the point of intersection of the discipline of the body and the control of the population' (Foucault 1980: 125), lend themselves therefore to 'an intensification of each individual's desire, for, in and over [her] body' (1980: 57).

In a postmodern age, feminism cannot afford to cling to the crumbling artifice of liberal humanist subjectivity and bounded identity. Those concepts have already failed us, and we should not regret the conditions of their disintegration but remind ourselves that it has been male subjectivity at the centre of power, male identity as the referent standard against which women are marked. The control of reproduction is no new battleground: from the man-midwives of the seventeenth century through to the genetic engineers of the future, men have consistently challenged women's physical and ontological centrality. The Father-God as origin is a dominant Western myth; and though NRTs may seem provisionally to recuperate that identity at the expense of women, the direction of the technologies involved seems to indicate that nothing can be taken as secure. Despite the Human Genome Project[16] where the desire to map boundaries is at its most fundamental, most recent and anticipated developments in biogenetics have signalled that what is taken, in popular culture, to be the basic unit of identity – the gene – is itself fully manipulable, interchangeable and artificially replicable. What NRTs can do, then, paradoxically, is to contest fundamentally the notion of identity as limit at the same time as they appear in some applications to reassert the woman-mother template. But in so far as they disrupt the concept of the maternal body as one and the same, they open up a space in which women can resituate themselves beyond the dichotomies of fixed identities, as occupying multiple subject positions.

The ethical enterprise lies in laying claim to that space, in refusing the assimilations demanded by phallocratic practice and insisting instead on both material and ontological heterogeneity. The aim is not to efface maternal desire, as Firestone supposed, but both to pluralise its expression and move beyond to pluralise feminine desire itself. That is not to say that feminists should uncritically welcome NRTs, and clearly we cannot ignore the harmful effects in the everyday lives of women. But what is needed there is the implementation of specific strategies of resistance to meet the specific techniques of abuse, and, moreover, a recognition that though the new technologies potentially speak to further extensions of male power, women are not simply passive victims in the face of scientific developments (Birke *et al.* 1990: 58–9). The realities of power are ever present, but they cannot be ascribed homogeneous meaning or intent, and nor are the relations of power beyond transformation. The exposure of indiscriminate developments of NRTs at the expense of women is one important aim for FINRRAGE and other campaigning groups, but a predominantly empirical basis for enquiry and intervention cannot adequately engage with discursive significance. Once that is taken into account – not, I would stress, as a separate sphere but as one which fully encompasses the material – then we have reason to hope that the ontological dislocations of the postmodern body may yet serve feminist ends.

Conclusion

> The search for a form of morality acceptable to everybody in the sense that everyone should submit to it, strikes me as catastrophic.
>
> (Foucault 1988: 253–4)

Although I have consistently had the ethical in mind, the approach that I have outlined makes no claims, and is not intended, to resolve the moral questions of how each of us should behave in concrete situations. I am not concerned to offer any pre-given programme of morally correct behaviour, nor even to suggest that questions of right and wrong can be finally determined. The issue rather has been to displace the dichotomy of true and false, good and bad, to show how those categories and others, both abstract and material, always necessarily leak into one another. That is not to claim that the deconstruction of existing paradigms for morality denies the need for certain issues to be ascribed differential value – there are always concrete decisions to make and some resolutions will be better than others – but rather it demands that we should give up the certain ground that has served to authorise our decisions.

The attempt to uncover a feminist ethic should be understood not as the quest for a superior standpoint from which to constitute a new morality representative of the feminine, nor yet as the aspiration for a set of values designed to promote the interests of women as women. What matters, on the contrary, is to resist all and any formalisation, and to make instead an open-ended commitment to a plurality of values that cannot be determined in advance. What will necessarily entail the feminist goal of valorising women is the deconstruction of the very meanings that have seemed to guarantee the moral status of the individual. It is not that concepts such as freedom, rationality and equality have no place at all, but that in order to enact an adequate response in a multiplicity of social relations, and to an irreducible diversity of individuals, those notions which work to elide differences must be displaced. The poststructuralist move to problematise all homogeneous categories, not least those proposed by binary sexual difference, undercuts all appeal to universal standards and calls instead for a fine and simultaneous awareness both of specificity and of the instability of boundaries and distinctions.

What I have described as the ethical moment, the only moment indeed to which a postmodernist recuperation of ethics can address itself, must precede the operation of morality as such, where that concept – if it is to have meaning at all – is understood not as the systemisation of rules of behaviour, but as no more than discrete instances of better or worse choice. In declining to provide a fully rational and supposedly objective foundation for morality external to and independent of the moral subject, but rather in asserting the futility of such an aspiration, I do not mean to imply that all behaviours are of equal value. What counts is the degree of reflexivity, the extent to which the actor is self-critical in her response to others. The ethical moment is a matter not of closure but of radical openness to the multiple possibilities for becoming. We are neither the one nor the other; neither the selfsame nor simply different. Rather, the requirement is that we should position ourselves among others, claiming no special authority, but without eschewing responsibility either. The difference of the binary, wherein such concepts of good and bad, right and wrong, themselves gain currency, collapses, not into indifference as so many critics of postmodernism have suggested, but into a multiplicity of differences which cannot be grasped in advance and which resist stable definition. It is above all an ethic of risk.

The fear, shared by many feminist theorists, is that the deconstruction of Enlightenment ideals amounts to the destruction of all possible value. In contradistinction, my claim is that that fear makes sense only within a model in which an ideal (albeit illusory) standard exists – for 'the good' or 'Truth', for example – that can be discovered by the exercise of rationality. Deconstruction concerns itself with how all foundational and universal claims are simply an effect of discourse, held in place by the naming and violent exclusion of difference. The yearning for the certainty of absolutes has resulted historically not in justice or equality or liberty, but in the denial of moral personhood to all those categories of living beings who cannot be identified in terms of the ideal standard. But once the binary of ideal/non-ideal has been displaced, once it is acknowledged that full and final definition is always deferred, it becomes possible to seek new constructions which no longer operate on the basis of exclusion. It is not the purpose of postmodernism to find ways to reinstate the terms of the Enlightenment, but nor is the task to destroy them. On a pragmatic level, negotiation with existing paradigms, as Spivak recommends, is always necessary, but what is important is that there is no single measure against which all claims are to be assessed. And by throwing into doubt the meaning of such terms as 'agency', 'identity', 'subjectivity' and 'autonomy', the dimensions of our ethical economies must be radically changed.

Given that traditional systems of morality are fundamentally reliant on the interplay of notions of sameness and difference, the problematisation of identity cannot but disrupt the strategies of justification operative within those models. If the subject, to use that term in a provisional sense, is always already shot through with otherness, then the conditions for the emergence of an ethics in themselves demand an openness to the encounter with the unmarked other, the other that is neither the same nor different. Where binary difference finally makes no difference but is simply another form of identity, *différance* makes all the difference. The singular voice of authority, guaranteed by the rationality of the unified and self-present one, is destabilised, at least revealed as contingent, at most as fragmented. Similarly, the illusion of order and intelligibility maintained by the displacement of disordered elements into the marked and feminised term is undermined by its own excess that escapes the binary. It is the spectre of otherness that returns to haunt the selfsame. So if identity, both in the sense of the self-contained, self-conscious subject and in terms of the sameness/difference between individuals will not hold, then we must ask what kind of ethical discourse could there be that was not constrained by those illusory boundaries.

As I outlined at the end of Chapter 3, the Derridean answer devolves precisely on the responsibility of facing the incalculable, of refusing the reliance on ideal or normative structures: 'Responsibility carries with it, and must do so, an essential excessiveness. It regulates itself neither on the principle of reason nor on any sort of accountancy' (Derrida 1991, 'Eating well': 108). The ethical, then, is inseparable from excessiveness; and moreover, as Derrida insists, though it is undecidable, its possibilities are nonetheless determined in 'strictly *defined* situations' (1988: 148). Now this focus on what is in Derridean terms primarily linguistic excess necessarily extends to the political and ethical project of the feminine, and to a consideration of the bioethics of the body. The corporeal economies which link the not-yet emergent feminine with the not-quite effaced body have been traced through Irigaray in particular, and I want to recall here that the logos, women and bodies are all compromised by their inherent leakiness. Just as the structure of the law – in Derrida's sense – has relied on the suppression and exclusion of its others, so too the feminine and the corporeal have been acknowledged only as the marked term of the masculine and the mind. What is at stake here is the modernist desire to establish impermeable absolutes, and that has necessarily involved fantasies of control – of words, of women and of the body. The ethics of modernity, then, far from responding to the incalculable, have operated to put in place just those normative values which effect control.

The bioethics which I have taken throughout as a focus for my critique are reliant on the implicit assumption both of a common identity and that the purpose of health care is to mitigate the disorders of the body. As a disciplinary practice in its own right, however, bioethics does much more than regulate the parameters of biomedical technologies: it is fully implicated in the inscription of the very body it seeks to describe, and ostensibly to protect. What I am suggesting, in contradistinction to the convention, is that what is really being protected is the illusory closure of a unified self. To forgo the myth of identity, to undo the binary of order/disorder must result in a very different ethic, then, in which normalisation would be meaningless. It is not only that the body is constituted in discourse rather than given as natural, but that it can never be fixed or sealed. The transgressive excess that health care attempts to counter is not peculiar to marginal bodies, but is an integral possibility of all bodies.

The dominant pattern of conventional bioethics as it has developed as a branch of applied philosophy has left no place for any discussion or problematisation of either the subject or the body itself. Where the body is scarcely considered at all but is taken simply as the gross material base of health-care practices, the subject is an issue only in so far as bioethics is concerned with who is to count as a moral agent. The privileging of patient autonomy as the appropriate goal of ethical practice amounts to little more than a narrow and overdetermined focus on consent. What is almost entirely absent from such models, in which it is implicit that the control of the body is the central point, is any space for an understanding of how the experience of illness or disability might itself constitute new subject positions not just resistant but excessive to the norms of the Western logos. The phenomenological account of subjectivity does at least in-corporate change, but it remains tied to an image of the ideal universal body. In both accounts, illness and disability are set against health in a binary model which posits them as disruptive but ultimately containable forces. But if, as I have shown, bodies themselves are not fixed, then we must see health care as entailing a great deal more than the preservation of body boundaries.

In the late twentieth century, the rapid development of an array of high-tech medical interventions, particularly in the area of procreation, has brought into crisis the purpose of health care. The possibilities are no longer simply those of corporeal normalisation, but, on the contrary, of the transgressive inter-changeability of body parts; the blurring of distinctions between life and death; the bypassing of generations in reproduction; the creation of genetically transformed individuals; and much else besides. But it is not that medical science has become detached from solid foundations and is now out of control, both materially and morally. Rather, it is that the relative technical sophistication of a postmodern age starkly underlines the *illusion* of control that has sustained medical knowledge from the start. The 'theory' of deconstruction and the practices of postmodern bioscience mesh together to dis-integrate the unified self, the gender binary, the normal body, and the ethics of sameness and difference. I am not suggesting that there is no place for the paradigms of the post-Enlightenment, but that they are no more than necessary fictions to be negotiated with caution and scepticism. A science and culture of boundaries generates an ethics of autonomy, of the proper, of rights and interests, and of contracts; an ethics of fixed limits rather than an ethics of the lived and changing body. It is moreover an ethics in which sexual difference is reduced to the binary exclusivity of the male/not-male pair.

What I have proposed, in contrast, is not the end of ethics but a radical rethinking of what might constitute the ethical moment. The modernist self-critique has stressed the need for a more relational, contextual and responsible morality – one that is often represented as, though not I think exhausted by, an ethics of care. I do not entirely reject that but want to go further, not to claim a superior truth, but to mark that that paradigm is no less contingent than others. As far as feminism is concerned, there is good reason to welcome any reconceptualisation which promises a more positive account of women, but postmodernists cannot remain indifferent to the underlying instability of the terms of the debate. What deconstruction has enabled us to do is to circumvent the irresolvable liberal feminist tension between gender specificity and gender impartiality. Where sexual difference is only the difference of the binary there is no escape from the inherent limitations of the operative categories, but the tracing of sexual difference 'beyond' the binary speaks to a multiplicity of differences in which all women might find a place. It is not my claim that poststructuralism/postmodernism inevitably yields such an outcome, but that it is the specifically feminist take-up of that problematic which opens up such possibilities. The fragmentation most usually associated with postmodernism and feared for its destructive potential is to be celebrated both for its shattering of masculinist certainties, and for the refusal to exclude the complication of fluid boundaries.

The deconstruction of binary dichotomies, those clear and distinct categories of difference which have marked the ambivalent relationship to the other who is both necessary and excluded, is the initial step of reinscribing the feminine in the ontological and epistemological framework. And if that framework were not just to encompass radical sexual difference but also embodied selves, then any expression of the ethical too must be rethought. The strand of postmodernist feminism that insists on the significance of embodiment turns away from the value-resistant and free-floating abstractions of an ultimately ir-responsive postmodernism, and asserts that it is not all immaterial. To be committed to any agenda to valorise women entails, then, both the deconstruction of exclusive and essential identities and the move to re-evaluate the body beyond biologistic, universalist and normative presuppositions. If women were no longer marginalised, no longer objectified in the symbolic and social order, no longer subjected to violence, both discursive and material, then the possibilities of ethical response would be reopened.

There must be no final closure on the question of ethics. Where a substantive field beckons, as it does in the case of bioethics, postmodernism declines to provide easy answers, but what it does make clear are the necessary preconditions for any adequate response to the diversity of relationships, and to the specificity of the dilemmas that inform health-care practice. The deconstruction of stable, homogeneous and hierarchical categories need not result in confusion and indistinction, but in an elaboration of differences and a sensitivity to change that demands precision and rigour. If the moral considerations which conventionally circumscribe good practice are to retain meaning at all, it is as an afterthought to the ethical moment. What matters, in bioethics, and more generally for the ethical affirmation of the feminine, is that an acceptance of the leakiness of bodies and boundaries speaks to the necessity of an open response. The other within the same is far more than a metaphor for the reproductive potential of women's bodies; it is an expression of the discursive interplay between all bodies and all subjects. Where modernist morality directs itself to the other as alien, as simply different, postmodernist feminism relocates the ethical moment as the response to the intimate other, never fully and finally separate, yet always non-identical in multiple ways to the self.

Notes

INTRODUCTION

1 It is important to note from the very beginning that my project makes historically and geopolitically limited claims. It does not, and cannot, speak for all women at all times, and indeed almost all generalisations, as I shall later show in the text, should be treated with caution. Nonetheless, as part of clearing the decks as it were, certain limiting generalisations are necessary at this stage.

2 The term 'provisionality' is used throughout in a postmodernist rather than Marxist sense. It should not be taken to imply any teleological process towards a final goal.

3 The term *bricoleur* originally derives from its use by Lévi-Strauss and is used to denote one who actively draws together disparate strands to produce new, and sometimes transgressive, meanings.

4 A glossary of abbreviations appears on pp. 244–5.

5 The so-called Hippocratic Oath promises mutual professional respect, beneficence, non-maleficence, the preservation of life, equal access to care and confidentiality.

6 Except where it is plainly debarred – in reference to Kant's work, for example, or sometimes that of Foucault – I have consistently used the pronoun 'she' to describe the moral actor. My purpose is both to provoke the inevitable tension that the concept of female moral agency generates within the supposed gender neutrality of the universal subject, and to flag the possibility of reconceiving and revalorising the feminine.

7 Irigaray's position is that throughout Western history the terms 'woman' and 'feminine' have existed not in their own right, but only as an adjunct of 'man' and 'masculine'. She looks forward nonetheless to a time when 'woman'/'feminine' will have independent meaning.

8 The issues outlined here are just those with which Liz Grosz engages at length in *Volatile Bodies* (1994) in order to establish a 'corporeal feminism' inseparable from the operation of sexual difference. Her concern is to flag, rather than develop, the epistemological implications of such a new perspective, while my own is to move forward in the specific area of ethics.

1 FABRICA(TIONS)

1 The notion of the 'one-sex' body which is said to underlie some contemporary anatomical representations is itself now a disputed discourse, but does seem to occupy a dominant position in the Renaissance and early modern period. See Laqueur (1990a), Tuana (1988, 1993) and Jacquart and Thomasset (1988) for a positive view of its importance.

2 Foucault was not entirely consistent in his understanding of the body, and this highly discursive approach should be set against his treatment in *The History of Sexuality*, volume 1, where he implies that the body might have some quasi-foundational anarchic truth.

3 The self-abusive behaviour of the thirteenth-century saint, Elizabeth of Spalbeck, graphically recorded by a contemporary in Ms Douce 114 (Horstmann 1885: 107–18) is a case in point. See also Bynum (1987) and Bell (1985) for similar biographies.

4 It is not that male bodies cannot be construed as similarly leaky, as, for example, in the form of unconstrained sexuality – the *spilling* of seed – but that what is understood as a matter of avoidable excess for the male is with the female intrinsic.

5 Fluidity is a central trope in Irigaray's early work, where it stands in a privileged relationship to female excess. See in particular 'Volume-fluidity' (1985a: 227–41). The male response 'finds everything flowing abhorrent' in that '[a]ll threaten to deform, propagate, evaporate, consume him, to flow out of him and into another who cannot be easily held on to' (1985a: 237). In 'The "mechanics" of fluids' (1985b, *This Sex Which Is Not One*: 106–18) Irigaray offers an explanation for the horror of fluidity when she asks rhetorically: 'what structuration of (the) language does not maintain a *complicity of long standing between rationality and a mechanics of solids alone?*'(1985b: 107).

6 This is not to say that in the modern period there are not many competing discourses of health which generate a variety of definitions and corresponding practices. What concerns me here is strictly the medical model, towards which biomedical ethics has in general orientated itself, in terms of both accommodation and challenge.

7 I use the term 'the medical model' to denote a specific sociological construct. It should not be taken to imply that other, albeit less dominant models, did not exist within the discipline of medicine.

8 I shall be discussing the nature of this choice and who makes it and why in Chapter 6.

9 It must be stressed again that my concern here is primarily with scientific discourse. For the complex reinscriptions of the links of both *femininity* and *masculinity* with nature in 'aesthetic' discourse, see Christine Battersby's argument in *Gender and Genius* (1989).

10 In an interesting thesis, Carroll Smith-Rosenberg suggests that in the context of nineteenth-century America, female hysteria represented a revolt against the disempowerment of women. The patients were both subject to control by others and exercised their own form of passive control by taking on the sick role. That contemporary doctors

saw the condition in moral terms is evidenced in the writings of S. Weir Mitchell, who warned that hysterical women had failed to develop 'rational endurance – [they] had early lost their power of self rule'; and Charles Lockwood who claimed that 'the poor sufferer is ... at the mercy of ... evil and unrestrained passions, appetites and morbid thoughts and impulses' (both quoted in Smith-Rosenberg 1984: 29).

Similar feminist analyses purport to explain a range of 'dieting' disorders not in terms of lack of control but of a resolute, and potentially self-destructive, effort to exercise a degree of self-determination in one's life. Orbach (1979), for example, explains anorexic conditions as a refusal to conform with the expectations of feminine sexuality.

11 For example, see Anne Fausto-Sterling (1992), *Myths of Gender* (passim); and Kathryn Pauly Morgan, 'Women and moral madness', (1988: 150–1) for a feminist overview. More specifically medical texts include Clayton *et al.*, *Gynaecology by Ten Teachers* wherein menstruation is consistently linked to emotional disturbance, even acts of violence (1980: 262).

12 The conventional medical texts in present-day use are hardly more sophisticated in their blatant bias against the female body. Consider these extracts from the section on 'The female urogenital triangle' in the 1990 edition of *Last's Anatomy*:

All the male formations and structures are present in the female, but *modified* greatly for functional reasons. The essential difference is the *failure* in the female of midline fusion of the genital folds. The male scrotum is *represented* by the labia majora of the vulva and the corpus spongiosum of the male urethra is *represented* by the labia minora and bulb of the vestibule.

The perineal membrane triangular ligament of the male is *represented* in the female by *only a narrow shelf ... Lacking* the rigid support of the *complete* perineal membrane of the male, the perineal body is more mobile in the female.
And on the female urethra:

There are a few *poorly developed* pit-like glands, said to be homogolous with the prostate, but bearing *no resemblance* to the structure of that gland.

(McMinn 1990: 412; emphases mine)

(I am grateful to Jocelyn Wogan-Browne for drawing this text to my attention.)

13 For medieval views of women's bodies as excessive, permeable and fissured, see Lochrie (1991).

14 An alternative and privileged explanation was that what was already perfect (male bodies) would not be likely to change into something less perfect (Maclean 1980: 39).

15 I use the term 'patriarchy', and its derivatives, with some caution, because as Spivak succinctly puts it: 'it is susceptible to biologistic,

naturalistic, and/or positivist-historical interpretations, and most often provides us with no more (and no less) than a place of accusation' (1987: 192, note 2). My primary understanding of patriarchy is of a system in which the dominant discourses privilege the male term as the norm or ideal, and which leads in turn to particular configurations of power.

16 Though objections may be raised with respect to the precise accuracy and adequacy of Foucault's historical claims here and elsewhere, I follow Gutting in seeing them as heuristic. Referring to the work on madness, Gutting writes:

> Foucault is not concerned with formulating exceptionless empirical generalizations from the historical data but with giving an overall characterization of a society's fundamental attitudes.... Such attitudes may well not be manifest in all texts and practices, and their existence can even be compatible with a variety of contrary tendencies.

(1989: 105)

17 See, for example, the General Household Survey (OPCS 1994), which highlights the trend for self-reported, limiting, longstanding illness to affect a higher proportion of females than males.

18 For a detailed analysis of how such a move operates with regard to the colonial state, see Price and Shildrick (1995).

19 Chapters 3 and 5 will explain and investigate this assertion in some detail.

2 FOUNDATIONS

1 I leave it to others, who are broadly sympathetic to the modernist framework, to give a more detailed critique of how such ethical terms are (mis)applied. See, for example, Bernard Williams, *Ethics and the Limits of Philosophy* (1985); Jonathan Dancy, *Moral Reasons* (1993); and Anne Maclean, *The Elimination of Morality* (1993).

2 Jean-Jacques Rousseau provides the clearest statement of a 'consequentialist' contract, but he is clear too that our entry into society generates rights within and duties to that society (1817, *Of the Social Contract*, esp. Bk 1: 55–7; trans. 1984).

3 'Duty is the necessity to act out of reverence for the law' (Paton 1961: 68). Kant's moral philosophy is most fully laid out in the *Groundwork of the Metaphysic of Morals*, first published in 1785. I refer to the Paton edition.

4 Downie and Calman, for example, see the person to be treated as self-determining and self-governing (1987: 53), though the extent of her agency *within* the health-care encounter is left unclear.

5 Alasdair MacIntyre has criticised medical ethics in particular as one area where 'the ideological function of the dominant conception of applied ethics masks transactions in which professional power and authority are being asserted in a way that will protect professional

autonomy from general moral scrutiny.' (1984, 'Does applied ethics rest on a mistake?': 498).

6 Jonathan Glover (1977), *Causing Death and Saving Lives*, chapter 5, for example, qualifies his utilitarian approach by insisting that autonomy must be incorporated as a preference.

7 Justice Cardozo in *Schloendorff* v. *Society of New York Hospital* (1914): 'Every human being of adult years and sound mind has a right to determine what shall be done with his own body.' See also *Natanson* v. *Kline* (Kan, 1960).

8 The benchmark case in English law is *Bolam* v. *Friern Hospital Management Committee* (1957) where McNair J. held that a doctor must act 'in accordance with a practice *accepted as proper by a responsible body of medical men* skilled in that art' (my emphasis). That this so-called professional standard of care applies to the giving of information and advice was confirmed in *Sidaway* v. *Board of Governors of Bethlem Royal Hospital* (1985) H.L. The majority judgment rejected both the (subjective) 'particular patient' and the (objective) 'prudent patient' test (by then current in some American state law) in favour of the Bolam test of how much and what information must be given to validate consent.

Even in the United States where the reasonable patient test is more commonly used, the standard set is an objective one, based on rational norms rather than one which takes account of the actual experience of particular patients.

9 In *The Treatise*, Hume firmly disputes the rationalist view of the authority of moral principles. His claim is that 'reason alone can never be a motive to any action . . . and can never oppose any passion in the direction of the will' (1962, 2,3,3: 125). See also Christine Battersby's *Gender and Genius* (1989) for an exposition of such counter-discourses.

3 FRACTURES

1 See *On the Basis of Morality* (Schopenhauer 1965: section 19).

2 Foucault's use of the term should not be elided with that used by Sartre and de Beauvoir, or even Lacan, where it has different connotations. The concept of the gaze was developed throughout Foucault's work, and denotes a constructive rather than antagonistic moment. It does not necessarily rely on an actual or hypothetical relationship with another, but, as I discussed in Chapter 1, can take the form of self surveillance. See *Birth of the Clinic* (1973: 8–9); *Discipline and Punish* (1977a: 198); *History of Sexuality*, vol. 1 (1979: 30); 'The eye of power' (1980, *Power/Knowledge*: 146–66) for the various forms it took.

3 See, in particular, Nancy Fraser's account in *Unruly Practices* (1989).

4 Genevieve Lloyd (1984), Jean Grimshaw (1986), Andrea Nye (1989), Janice Moulton (1989) and Moira Gatens (1991) are among the many who have addressed this issue with varying degrees of sophistication.

5 One is reminded here of the similar process by which medieval male sainthood was negotiated (Bynum 1987).

6 Lloyd's essay is reprinted here in Garry and Pearsall (eds) (1989). The same ideas are more fully developed in her own book *The Man of Reason* (1984).

7 Sartre's views on women are rarely given directly, but his frequent references to the 'feminine', particularly as they develop in Part 4 of *Being and Nothingness* (1958), seem to justify de Beauvoir's subsequent identification of woman with the pure Other (de Beauvoir 1968: 8). Like Sartre, de Beauvoir opposes transcendence and immanence, and genders them as masculine and feminine categories respectively. In her view, nonetheless, *women* are able to become subjects by transcending the materiality of the female body.

8 Where the potential for a newly conceived ethics has been taken up by some male commentators – as, for example, in work by Zygmunt Bauman (1993) – it is as an enterprise that betrays no gender awareness.

9 The term *différance* was first introduced in 1968 by Derrida in a lecture of the same name, subsequently reprinted in *Speech and Phenomena* (1973). It has since appeared in many manifestations and under other names, such as 'gram', 'trace', 'supplement', 'pharmakon', 'hymen' – those things which Derrida calls the undecidables (1981a: 43). My remarks here relate to its early use in such texts as *Of Grammatology* (1976).

10 The epistemic confusion about sex and gender is clearly exemplified in a newspaper report (*Guardian*, 29 October 1992) entitled 'Sex-test row hits Olympics'. It outlines how what is then named as the *femininity* test demanded of Olympic participants can take various forms focused on either genital appearance, genetic make-up or hormonal distribution. It is unclear, however, whether the aim of each test, which is to detect unfair 'male' physiological advantage in 'female' competitors, must rely on some notion of the foundational truth of either sex or gender. Is a woman carrying an unexpressed male gene more or less female than a woman receiving injected male hormone supplements? The only constant seems to be that a 'real' woman, however she is constructed, is at a physiological disadvantage to men.

11 See Sarah Lucia Hoagland, '"Femininity", resistance and sabotage' (1986: 78). Also Naomi Schor, 'Dreaming dissymmetry' (1989: 47).

12 It is worth noting, however, that lingering notions of essence remain in familiar verbal constructs like 'always already'. Diana Fuss (1989) suggests, strictly in line with the poststructuralist agenda, that essence should be not so much denied as displaced.

4 FEMINIST ETHICS

1 There are of course other models of autonomy, notably a situationist one, which do not entail the features I describe here. The dominant discourse of health-care ethics has little place for them.

2 See, for example, Lorraine Code (1988), 'Experience, knowledge and responsibility'; Ann Ferguson (1989), 'A feminist aspect theory of the self'; and Andrea Nye (1989), *Feminist Theories and the Philosophies of Man*.

3 I do not subscribe, however, to the view that mutual realisation necessarily devolves from the *experiential* connection between women and nurturance. The attempt to sidestep essentialism seems bound to fail, at least partially, unless the biological body itself is problematised as a discursive construction. For a committed but 'simple' view of the link between realisation and nurturance, see, however, Caroline Whitbeck (1989), 'A different reality: feminist ontology'. Like Gilligan, Whitbeck would be classed as a difference theorist in its Anglo-American sense; but here the term marks a closure rather than the opening up of possibilities – associated in poststructuralism both with the play of differences, and with the recuperation of sexual difference attempted most notably by Luce Irigaray.

4 It is the feminist political agenda of valorising women that will determine when a moment of/for resistance might occur. Gayatri Spivak, for example, habitually insists on the necessity to realise such moments.

5 In Chapter 6 I give an extended analysis of how issues of access to assisted reproduction – that is, to donor insemination, *in vitro* fertilisation, and to other technologically managed programmes – can be reconstructed in the light of such a poststructuralist critique.

6 Habermas (1984) sees modern society as characterised by the separation of the distinct areas of lifeworld and system. The lifeworld denotes that everyday context within which individuals and groups are socially integrated, both in terms of the domestic sphere of the family, and through political participation and debate. In contrast, the system is the sphere of power and money, of the modern administrative state and the capitalist economy. I understand it to be equivalent to what Porter means by the public sphere.

5 FEMINIST THEORY AND POSTMODERNISM

1 Yet again I want to flag very clearly that my remarks are localised within the Western European and Anglo-American context.

2 My reference to 'liberal feminist' implies not simply a categorical position that might be capitalised as Liberal Feminism (which concerns itself primarily with the attainment of equality for women), but rather a whole range of feminisms which are situated in terms of the humanist project. Thus the conventional denominators of liberal, radical and socialist/Marxist feminism are implicated equally in an uncritical stance towards those things – most specifically here stable subjectivity – that postmodernist feminism contests.

3 See, in particular, Gayatri Spivak's essay 'Can the subaltern speak?' in *In Other Worlds* (1988).

4 I have Foucault and Derrida most particularly in mind here. The claim would not necessarily hold for Lacanian analytics, in so far as the phallus as transcendental signifier is (mis)identified in fantasy with the penis, but I am by no means certain that Lacan can be named as a poststructuralist.

5 See the two introductory chapters of *Feminine Sexuality* (Mitchell and Rose 1982) for a summary of the relevant Lacanian concepts.

6 Though Haraway is certainly distanced from the humanist standpoint theory, she has endorsed, nonetheless, a postmodern version of sorts which relies on 'partial, locatable, critical knowledges' (1988, 'Situated knowledges': 584). She goes on, however, to insist that no standpoint is ever innocent, because 'we are not immediately present to ourselves' (ibid.).

7 'Choreographies: an interview with Jacques Derrida' was conducted by Christie McDonald and first appeared in the journal *Diacritics*, 12 (Summer 1982): 67–76. It was reprinted in *The Ear of the Other* (1985a), to which edition all subsequent page numbers refer.

8 Although Derrida is prepared to acknowledge, and even celebrate, 'the enormous deconstructive import of the feminine as an uprooting of our phallogocentric culture' (Kearney 1984, 'Deconstruction and the Other': 121), his approbation does not usually extend to feminism. See, for example, the article 'Deconstruction in America' in *Critical Exchange 17* where Derrida states: 'I would say that deconstruction is deconstruction of feminism, from the start, in so far as feminism is a form ... of phallogocentrism among others' (1985b: 30–1).

9 This theme is developed at length in 'Plato's *Hystera*' in *Speculum of the Other Woman* (1985a). See also 'Cosi Fan Tutti' in *This Sex Which Is Not One* (1985b: 86–106).

10 My use of this phrase derives from Hélène Cixous's famous metaphor in 'Sorties' (1987, *The Newly Born Woman*: 94), which captures the notion of feminine writing both as intrinsically intertwined with breast-milk and as invisible within the male symbolic.

11 In response to my speculation, made at a workshop at University of Warwick, May 1993, Derrida claimed that 'blended' was a poor translation of the word which he had used in his original French answer to Christie McDonald's question. As, however, 'Choreographies' has appeared for many years *only* in English, I would maintain that he bears some responsibility for the publication of that specific translation. It is no surprise that he should wish now to repudiate it.

12 Leder, however, generally prefers to see others in terms of mutuality and co-transcendence rather than as intrinsically hostile.

13 Young specifies, in fact, that it is young adult males who see the body as unchanging (1984: 56).

14 In more recent work – and notably *Volatile Bodies* – Liz Grosz has moved strongly towards a recuperation of the materiality of the corporeal, both in Irigaray, and for herself. But as she stresses: '[bodies] are materialities that are uncontainable in physicalist terms alone' (1994: xi).

15 Irigaray's later work is far more problematic with respect to the charge of essentialism, and her deployment of sexual difference has seemed increasingly to suggest certain pre-given and determinant qualities of the feminine. But given that I am concerned not to explicate the Irigarayan opus, but to make use of some of her ideas, I make no apology for choosing what suits my own ends, even though those particular ideas may have evolved in a quite different way. I am, in other words, not content to accept the authority of the author.

6 LEAKS AND FLOWS

1 Where infection is implicated, it may well be that heterosexual women are at greater risk, but in any case it should be remembered that as much as 65 per cent of lesbians have been heterosexually active at some time (Ettorre 1980: 86). Further, some forms of disablement carry a greater risk of infection leading to infertility.

2 See Judith Lorber (1989: 23) for an analysis of why fertile women might agree to such procedures.

3 The judgment in *R.* v. *Ethical Committee of St Mary's Hospital (Manchester), ex parte H* (1988) provided a rare insight into the operation of – at that point – unofficial, but by no means uncommon, access restrictions. In the absence of legally binding criteria, individual providers of AR have been able to set their own terms for treatment.

4 The term was used throughout the British press during March 1991 following reports that BPAS had provided DI to at least three women, of whom none had ever had a sexual relationship with a man.

5 Even in those early days the potential for AI to be used as a mechanism of social control was apparent. See, for example, Herbert Brewer's article 'Eutelegenesis', published in July 1935: 121–6.

6 See, for example, the report 'Wish to avoid sex "may hide neurosis"' in the *Guardian,* 12 March 1991.

7 In March 1991 the right-wing Conservative MP Dame Jill Knight was widely quoted as saying of virgin mothers: 'to deliberately make a woman pregnant who obviously has none of the natural feelings about the matter I think is irresponsible'. (See, for example, the *Guardian,* 12 March 1991.)

8 Mill's famous formulation in 'On liberty' (Warnock 1979: 135) establishes the basis for this view.

9 But note that this is a potentially dangerous argument for feminists to pursue, in that such a right may swiftly devolve into the notion of consortium whereby women would once again lose control of their own fertility. What is intended, for example in the UN *Universal Declaration of Human Rights* (1948, Article 16, Pt 1), as a *liberty* right – meaning that the right 'to found a family' should not be interfered with – may be taken as a *claim* right exercised by men against women.

10 FINRRAGE is the acronym for Feminist International Network of Resistance to Reproductive and Genetic Engineering, a group formed

in July 1985 at the Women's Emergency Conference on NRTs held in Vallinge, Sweden. The name is explicitly intended to suggest that NRTs are harmful to women and should be seen in almost wholly negative terms (Spallone and Steinberg 1987: 2). The opening statement of the FINRRAGE resolution reads:

> We women ... declare that the female body, with its unique capacity for creating human life, is being expropriated and dissected as raw material for the technological production of human beings. For us women, for nature, and for the exploited peoples of the world, this development is a declaration of war. Genetic and reproductive engineering is another attempt to end self-determination over our bodies.
>
> (Reported in Spallone and Steinberg 1987: 211)

11 The preferred use of IVF holds true even when the more simple form of it is ineffective and micro-injection of the sperm directly into the ovum is indicated. The procedure is still under development and has at present an extremely poor success rate (Human Fertilisation and Embryology Authority Annual Report 1993).

12 The Warnock Committe, for example, approved the use of IVF for male infertility because of its 'social benefit' in leading to a baby that is the genetic offspring of both partners (Warnock Report 1984: 32, section 5.9).

13 References are too numerous to list individually. The journal *Issues in Reproductive and Genetic Engineering* is a consistent source for each category of objection. Relevant books and articles appearing elsewhere tend to be less committed a priori to a negative view of NRTs, but nonetheless reiterate many of the same issues. See, for example: Michelle Stanworth (ed.), *Reproductive Technologies. Gender, Motherhood and Medicine* (1987); Christine Overall (ed.), *The Future of Human Reproduction* (1989); Jocelynne A. Scutt (ed.), *The Baby Machine: Reproductive Technology and the Commercialisation of Motherhood* (1990); Lynda Birke *et al. Tomorrow's Child: Reproductive Technologies in the Nineties* (1990); Ruth S. Chadwick, *Ethics, Reproduction and Genetic Control* (1992); and various articles appearing in *Hypatia*, particularly those in the issue entitled 'Ethics and reproduction' (Fall 1989, vol. 4, 3).

14 The misapprehension that radical feminism necessarily posits an essential female nature and sexuality may explain much of the mistrust between radical and postmodernist feminists. The traffic in scepticism is not, however, all one way, and those radical feminists who do take the FINRRAGE line appear hostile to any insights generated by postmodernism. The journal *Issues in Reproduction and Genetic Engineering*, which is closely associated with FINRRAGE, is extremely reluctant to publish any material coming from a postmodernist stance.

15 See, for example, *Power/Knowledge*: 'there are no relations of power without resistances; the latter are all the more real and effective because they are formed right at the point where relations of power are exercised' (Foucault 1980: 142).

16 The Human Genome Project is a multi-billion-dollar international project which aims to sequence all the DNA that occurs in human chromosomes. The resulting map is intended to enable an understanding of how human characteristics are inherited and how genetic diseases are passed on. For a critical appraisal, see Hubbard and Wald (1993).

Bibliography

The date given in each case refers only to the particular edition cited, and may not be the original date of publication.

Althusser, Louis (1971) 'Ideology and ideological state apparatuses', in *Lenin and Philosophy*, London: New Left Books.

Aristotle (1953) *De generatione animalium*, trans. A.L. Peck, London: Heinemann.

——(1961) *Metaphysics*, ed. and trans. John Warrington, London: Dent.

Armstrong, David (1983) *The Political Anatomy of the Body: Medical Knowledge in Britain in the Twentieth Century*, Cambridge: Cambridge University Press.

Bartky, Sandra Lee (1988) 'Foucault, femininity and patriarchal power', in Irene Diamond and Lee Quinby (eds) *Feminism and Foucault: Reflections on Resistance*, Boston: Northeastern University Press.

Battersby, Christine (1989) *Gender and Genius*, London: The Women's Press.

Bauman, Zygmunt (1993) *Postmodern Ethics*, Oxford: Blackwell.

Beauchamp, Tom and Childress, James (1983) *Principles of Biomedical Ethics*, Oxford: Oxford University Press.

Bell, Rudolph (1985) *Holy Anorexia*, Chicago: University of Chicago Press.

Benhabib, Seyla (1986) 'The generalized and concrete other: the Kohlberg–Gilligan controversy and feminist theory', *Praxis International* 5 (4): 402–25.

Berengario, Jacopo (1959) *A Short Introduction to Anatomy, Isagogae Breves*, trans. L.R. Lind with Anatomical Notes by P.G. Roofe, Chicago: University of Chicago Press.

Berg, Maggie (1991) 'Luce Irigaray's "Contradictions": poststructuralism and feminism', *Signs* 17 (1): 50–70.

Biology and Gender Study Group (1988) 'The importance of feminist critique for contemporary cell biology', *Hypatia* 3 (2): 61–75.

Birenbaum-Comeli, D. (1995) 'Maternal smoking during pregnancy: social, medical and legal perspectives on the conception of a human being', *Health Care International for Women* 16 (1): 57–73.

Birke, Lynda, Himmelweit, Susan and Vines, Gail (1990) *Tomorrow's Child: Reproductive Technologies in the Nineties*, London: Virago.

Bolam v *Friern Hospital Management Committee* (1957) 2 All ER 118.

Bordo, Susan (1990) 'Reading the slender body', in Mary Jacobus *et al.* (eds). *Body/Politics: Women and the Discourses of Science*, London, Routledge.

Boston Women's Health Book Collective (1976) *Our Bodies, Ourselves*, 2nd edn, New York: Simon & Schuster.

——(1978) *Our Bodies, Ourselves*, British edn, ed. Angela Phillips and Jill Rakusen, London: Penguin.

Braidotti, Rosi 1987) 'Envy: or with your brains and my looks', in Alice Jardine and Paul Smith (eds) *Men in Feminism*, London: Methuen.

——(1989a) 'Organs without bodies', *differences* 1 (1): 147–61.

——(1989b) 'The politics of ontological difference', in Teresa Brennan (ed.) *Between Feminism and Psychoanalysis*, London: Routledge.

——(1991a) *Patterns of Dissonance*, Cambridge: Polity Press.

——(1991b) 'On contemporary medical pornography', *Tijdschrift voor Vrouwenstudies* 47 (12, 3): 356–71.

Brewer, Herbert (1935) 'Eutelegenesis', *The Eugenics Review* xxvii: 121–6.

Brody, Barach A. (1990) 'Quality of scholarship in bioethics', *Journal of Medicine and Philosophy* 15: 161–78.

Brown, Wendy (1991) 'Feminist hesitations, postmodern exposures', *differences* 3 (1): 63–84.

Butler, Judith (1990) *Gender Trouble: Feminism and the Subversion of Identity*, London: Routledge.

——(1991) 'Imitation and gender insubordination', in Diana Fuss (ed.) *Inside/Out: Lesbian Theories, Gay Theories*, London: Routledge.

——(1992) 'Contingent foundations: feminism and the question of "postmodernism"', in Judith Butler and Joan W. Scott (eds) *Feminists Theorize the Political*, London: Routledge.

——(1993) *Bodies that Matter: On the Discursive Limits of "Sex"*, London: Routledge.

Butler, Judith and Scott, Joan W. (eds) (1992) *Feminists Theorize the Political*, London: Routledge.

Bynum, Caroline Walker (1987) *Holy Fast and Holy Feast: the Religious Significance of Food to Medieval Women*, Cambridge: Cambridge University Press.

Callahan, J.C. and Knight, J.W. (1992) 'Women, fetuses, medicine, and the law', in Helen Bequaert Holmes and Laura M. Purdy (eds) *Feminist Perspectives in Medical Ethics*, Bloomington: Indiana University Press.

Chadwick, Ruth S. (ed.) (1992) *Ethics, Reproduction and Genetic Control*, 2nd edn, London: Routledge.

Chanter, Tina (1995) *Ethics of Eros: Irigaray's Rewriting of the Philosophers*, London: Routledge.

Cixous, Hélène (1987) 'Sorties: out and out: attacks/ways out/forays', in Hélène Cixous and Catherine Clément *The Newly Born Woman*, trans. Betsy Wing, Manchester: Manchester University Press.

Clayton, S.G., Lewis, T.L.T. and Pinker, G. (eds) (1980) *Gynaecology by Ten Teachers*, London: Edward Arnold.

Code, Lorraine (1988) 'Experience, knowledge and responsibility' in M. Griffiths and M. Whitford (eds) *Feminist Perspectives in Philosophy*, London: Macmillan.

——(1992) 'Must a feminist be a relativist after all?' in Maja Pellikaan-Engel (ed.) *Against Patriarchal Thinking*, Amsterdam: VU University Press.

Code, Lorraine, Mullett, Sheila and Overall, Christine (eds) (1988) *Feminist Perspectives: Philosophical Essays on Method and Morals*, Toronto: University of Toronto Press.

Corea, Gena (1988) *The Mother Machine: Reproductive Technologies from Artificial Insemination to Artificial Wombs*, London: The Women's Press.

Cornell, Drucilla (1991) *Beyond Accommodation: Ethical Feminism, Deconstruction, and the Law*, London: Routledge.

Council for Science and Society (1984) *Human Procreation: Ethical Aspects of the New Techniques*, Oxford: Oxford University Press.

Daly, Mary (1979) *Gyn/Ecology: the Metaethics of Radical Feminism*, London: Women's Press.

Dancy, Jonathan (1993) *Moral Reasons*, Oxford: Blackwell.

de Beauvoir, Simone (1968) *Nature of the Second Sex*, originally *The Second Sex*, vol. 1, trans. H.M. Parshley, London: New English Library.

de Graaf, Regnerus (1672) *De mulierum organis generationi inservientibus*, Leiden: Haak.

de Lauretis, Teresa (1987) 'The rhetoric of violence', in *Technologies of Gender: Essays on Theory, Film and Fiction*, London: Macmillan.

—— (ed.) (1988) *Feminist Studies/Critical Studies*, London: Macmillan.

de Wit, Cynthia and Corea, Gena (1990) 'Current developments and issues: birth regulation', *Issues in Reproductive and Genetic Engineering* 3 (1): 51–70.

Deleuze, G. and Guattari, F. (1984) *Anti-Oedipus: Capitalism and Schizophrenia*, trans. R. Hurley, M Seem and H.R. Lane, London: Athlone.

Derrida, Jacques (1973) *Speech and Phenomena*, trans. David Allison, Evanston, IL: Northwestern University Press.

——(1976) *Of Grammatology*, with 'Preface' and trans. Gayatri Chakravorty Spivak, Baltimore, MD: Johns Hopkins University Press.

——(1979) *Spurs: Nietzsche's Styles*, trans. Barbara Harlow, Chicago: University of Chicago Press.

——(1981a) *Dissemination*, trans. Barbara Johnson, Chicago: University of Chicago Press.

——(1981b) *Positions*, trans. Alan Bass, London: Athlone Press.

——(1982) *Margins of Philosophy*, trans. Alan Bass, Brighton: Harvester.

——(1985a) 'Choreographies: an interview with Jacques Derrida', ed. and trans. Christie V. McDonald, in *The Ear of the Other*, Lincoln: University of Nebraska Press.

——(1985b) 'Deconstruction in America', *Critical Exchange* 17: 1–33.

——(1987) 'Women in the beehive: a seminar with Jacques Derrida', in Alice Jardine and Paul Smith (eds) *Men in Feminism*, London: Methuen.

——(1988) *Limited Inc*, ed. Gerald Graff, Evanston, IL: Northwestern University Press.

——(1991a) 'Geschlecht: sexual difference, ontological difference', trans. Reuben Berbezdivin, in Peggy Kamuf (ed.) *A Derrida Reader: Between the Blinds*, London: Harvester Wheatsheaf.

——(1991b) '"Eating well", or the calculation of the subject: an interview with Jacques Derrida', in Eduardo Cadava, Peter Connor and Jean-Luc Nancy (eds) *Who Comes After the Subject?* London: Routledge.

Descartes, René (1962) *A Discourse on Method*, ed. A.D. Lindsay, London: J.M. Dent.

Diprose, Rosalyn (1991) 'A "genethics" that makes sense' in R. Diprose and R. Ferrell (eds) *Cartographies: Poststructuralism and the Mapping of Bodies and Spaces*, Sydney: Allen & Unwin.

——(1994) *The Bodies of Women: Ethics, Embodiment and Sexual Difference*, London: Routledge.

Diprose, Rosalyn and Ferrell, Robyn (eds) (1991), *Cartographies: Poststructuralism and the Mapping of Bodies and Spaces*, Sydney: Allen & Unwin.

DLA 580 (1993) Disability Living Allowance Claim Pack, Benefits Agency.

Downie, R.S. and Calman, K.C. (1987) *Healthy Respect*, London: Faber & Faber.

Draper, Heather (1993) 'Women, forced caesarians and antenatal responsibilities', in Feminist Legal Research Unit, *Body Politics: Control versus Freedom*, University of Liverpool: Faculty of Law.

Dundas-Todd, A. (1989) *Intimate Adversaries*, Philadelphia: University of Pennsylvania Press.

Dworkin, Gerald (1976) 'Paternalism' in S. Gorowitz (ed.) *Moral Problems in Medicine*, Englewood Cliffs, NJ: Prentice-Hall.

Dworkin, Ronald (1984) 'Rights as trumps', in Jeremy Waldron (ed.) *Theories of Rights*, Oxford: Oxford University Press.

Eisenstein, Zillah (1989) *The Female Body and the Law*, Berkeley: University of California Press.

Engelhardt, H.T. (1986) *The Foundations of Bioethics*, Oxford: Oxford University Press.

Ettorre, E.M. (1980) *Lesbians, Women and Society*, London: Routledge & Kegan Paul.

Faulder, Caroline (1985) *Whose Body is It? The Troubling Issue of Informed Consent*, London: Virago.

Fausto-Sterling, Anne (1992) *Myths of Gender: Biological Theories about Women and Men*, New York: Basic Books.

Ferguson, Ann (1989) 'A feminist aspect theory of the self', in A. Garry and M. Pearsall (eds) *Women, Knowledge and Reality*, London: Unwin Hyman.

Feversham Committee (1960) *Report of the Departmental Committee on Human Artificial Insemination*, Cmnd 1105, London: HMSO.

Firestone, Shulamith (1979) *The Dialectic of Sex*, London: Women's Press.

Flax, Jane (1992) 'The end of innocence', in Judith Butler and Joan W. Scott (eds) *Feminists Theorize the Political*, London: Routledge.

Foucault, Michel (1972) *The Archaeology of Knowledge*, trans. A. Sheridan, London: Tavistock.

——(1973) *The Birth of the Clinic: an Archaeology of Medical Perception*, trans. A. Sheridan, London: Tavistock.

——(1977a) *Discipline and Punish: the Birth of the Prison*, trans. A. Sheridan, London: Allen Lane.

——(1977b) 'Nietzsche, genealogy, history' in Donald Bouchard (ed.) *Language, Counter-Memory, Practice: Selected Essays and Interviews*, Ithaca, NY: Cornell University Press.

——(1979) *The History of Sexuality*, vol.1, trans. R. Hurley, London: Allen Lane.

——(1980) *Power/Knowledge: Selected Interviews and Other Writings, 1972–77*, ed. Colin Gordon, Brighton: Harvester Press.

——(1982) 'The subject and power', an afterword to H. Dreyfus and P. Rabinow *Michel Foucault: Beyond Structuralism and Hermeneutics,* Chicago: Chicago University Press.

——(1985a) 'Sexuality and solitude', in M. Blonsky (ed.) *On Signs*, Baltimore, MD: Johns Hopkins University Press.

——(1985b) *The Use of Pleasure*, trans. R. Hurley, Harmondsworth: Penguin.

——(1986) *The Care of the Self*, trans. R. Hurley, Harmondsworth: Penguin.

——(1988) *Politics, Philosophy, Culture: Interviews and Other Writings 1977–1984*, ed. Lawrence D. Kritzman, London: Routledge.

Fox, Nicholas J. (1993) *Postmodernism, Sociology and Health*, Buckingham: Open University Press.

Fraser, Nancy (1989) *Unruly Practices: Power, Discourse and Gender in Contemporary Social Theory*, Cambridge: Polity Press.

Fuss, Diana (1989) *Essentially Speaking: Feminism, Nature and Difference*, London: Routledge.

Gadow, Sally (1980) 'Body and self: a dialectic', *Journal of Medicine and Philosophy* 5 (3): 172–85.

Galen (1968) *De usu partium*, trans. M.T. May, Ithaca, NY: Cornell University Press.

——(1992) *De semine*, trans. Phillip de Lacy, Berlin: Akademie Verlag.

Garry, Ann and Pearsall, Marilyn (eds) (1989) *Women, Knowledge and Reality*, London: Unwin Hyman.

Gatens, Moira (1991) *Feminism and Philosophy: Perspectives on Difference and Equality*, Cambridge: Polity Press.

Gilligan, Carol (1982) *In a Different Voice: Psychological Theory and Women's Development*, Cambridge, MA: Harvard University Press.

Gillon, Ranaan (1985) *Philosophical Medical Ethics*, Chichester: John Wiley.

—— (ed.) (1994) *Principles of Health Care Ethics*, Chichester: John Wiley.

Glover, Jonathan (1977) *Causing Death and Saving Lives*, London: Penguin Books.

Golombok, Susan and Rust, John (1986) 'The Warnock Report and single women: what about the children?, *Journal of Medical Ethics* 12: 182.

Graham, Hilary (1993) 'Social divisions in caring', *Women's Studies International Forum* 16 (5): 461–70.

Graham, Hilary and Oakley, Anne (1986) 'Competing ideologies of reproduction: medical and maternal perspectives on pregnancy', in C. Currer and M. Stacey (eds) *Concepts of Health, Illness and Disease*, Leamington Spa: Berg.

Griffin, Susan (1980) *Woman and Nature: the Roaring Inside Her*, New York: Harper Colophon.

Griffiths, Morwenna and Whitford, Margaret (eds) (1988) *Feminist Perspectives in Philosophy*, London: Macmillan.

Grimshaw, Jean (1986) *Feminist Philosophers: Women's Perspectives on Philosophical Traditions*, Brighton: Wheatsheaf.

Grosz, Elizabeth (1989) *Sexual Subversions: Three French Feminists*, Sydney: Allen & Unwin.

——(1990) 'Contemporary theories of power and subjectivity', in Sneja Gunew (ed.) *Feminist Knowledge: Critique and Construct*, London: Routledge.

——(1994) *Volatile Bodies: Towards a Corporeal Feminism*, London: Routledge.

Guardian (1991) 'Wish to avoid sex "may hide neurosis"', 12 March (Manchester edn).

——(1992) 'Sex-test row hits Olympics', 29 October (Manchester edn).

Gutting, Gary (1989) *Michel Foucault's Archaeology of Scientific Reason*, Cambridge: Cambridge University Press.

Habermas, Jurgen (1984) *Theory of Communicative Action*, vol.1, Boston: Beacon Press.

Haraway, Donna (1988) 'Situated knowledges: the science question in feminism and the privilege of partial perspectives', *Feminist Studies* 14 (3): 575–99.

——(1989) 'The biopolitics of postmodern bodies', *differences* 1 (1): 3–43.

——(1990) 'A manifesto for cyborgs: science, technology and socialist feminism in the 1980s', reprinted in Linda J. Nicholson (ed.) *Feminism/Postmodernism*, London: Routledge.

Harding, Sandra (1986) 'The instability of the analytic categories of feminist theory', *Signs: Journal of Women in Culture and Society* 11 (4): 645–65.

Hartsock, Nancy (1983) 'The feminist standpoint: developing the ground for a specifically feminist historical materialism', in Sandra Harding and Merrill B. Hintikka (eds) *Discovering Reality*, Dordrecht: D. Reidel.

——(1990) 'Foucault on power: a theory for women?', in Linda J. Nicholson (ed.) *Feminism/Postmodernism*, London: Routledge.

Hartsoeker, Nicolaus (1694) *Essai de diotropique*, Paris: Anisson.

Hekman, Susan J. (1990) *Gender and Knowledge: Elements of a Postmodern Feminism*, Cambridge: Polity Press.

Hirsch, Marianne and Keller, Evelyn Fox (eds) (1990) *Conflicts in Feminism,* London: Routledge.

Hoagland, Sarah Lucia (1986) '"Femininity", resistance and sabotage', in Marilyn Pearsall (ed.) *Women and Values*, Belmont, CA: Wadsworth.

Holmes, Helen Bequaert and Purdy, Laura M. (eds) (1992) *Feminist Perspectives in Medical Ethics*, Bloomington: Indiana University Press.

Holmes, Robert (1990) 'The limited relevance of analytic ethics to the problems of bioethics', *Journal of Medicine and Philosophy* 15: 143–59.

Horstmann, C. (1885) 'Prosalegenda', in R.P. Wulker (ed.) *Anglia VIII*, Halle a.S: Max Niemayer.

Hubbard, R. and Wald, E. (1993) *Exploding the Gene Myth*, Boston: Beacon Press.

Human Fertilisation and Embryology Authority (n.d.) *Annual Report 1993*, London: HFEA.

Hume, David (1962) *A Treatise of Human Nature*, ed. A.D. Lindsay, London: J.M. Dent.

Hursthouse, Rosalind (1987) *Beginning Lives,* Oxford: Blackwell.

Ingelfinger, F.J. (1980) 'Arrogance', *New England Journal of Medicine* 303: 1507–11.

Irigaray, Luce (1985a) *Speculum of the Other Woman*, trans. Gillian C. Gill, Ithaca, NY: Cornell University Press.

——(1985b) *This Sex Which Is Not One*, trans. Catherine Porter, New York: Cornell University Press.

——(1993a) *An Ethics of Sexual Difference*, trans. Carolyn Burke and Gillian C. Gill, London: Athlone Press.

——(1993b) 'On the maternal order' in *Je, Tu, Nous: Toward a Culture of Difference*, trans. Alison Martin, London: Routledge.

Jacobus, Mary (1990) 'In parenthesis: immaculate conceptions and female desire', in Mary Jacobus, Evelyn Fox Keller and Sally Shuttleworth (eds) *Body/Politics: Women and the Discourses of Science*, London: Routledge.

Jacobus, Mary, Keller, Evelyn Fox and Shuttleworth, Sally (eds) (1990) *Body/Politics: Women and the Discourses of Science*, London: Routledge.

Jacquart, Danielle and Thomasset, Claude (1988) *Sexuality and Medicine in the Middle Ages*, Cambridge: Polity Press.

Jardine, Alice (1985) *Gynesis: Configurations of Woman and Modernity*, Ithaca, NY: Cornell University Press.

Jordan, June (1989) 'Report from the Bahamas', in *Moving Towards Home: Political Essays*, London: Virago.

Jordanova, Ludmilla (1980) 'Natural facts: a historical perspective on science and sexuality' in C. MacCormack and M. Strathern (eds) *Nature, Culture and Gender*, Cambridge: Cambridge University Press.

——(1989) *Sexual Visions: Images of Gender in Science and Medicine between the Eighteenth and Twentieth Centuries*, London: Harvester Wheatsheaf.

Kant, Immanuel (1981) *Observations on the Feeling of the Beautiful and the Sublime*, trans. T.J. Goldthwait, Berkeley: University of California Press.

Kaplan, Ann E. (1992) *Motherhood and Representation*, London: Routledge.

Kearney, Richard (1984) 'Deconstruction and the Other' in *Dialogues with Contemporary Continental Thinkers*, Manchester: Manchester University Press.

Kennedy, Ian and Grubb, Andrew (1994) *Medical Law: Text with Materials*, London: Butterworths.

Kirejczyk, Marta (1992) 'New Reproductive Technologies: feminist discourse, gender and social entrenchment of *in vitro* fertilization in the Netherlands', unpublished paper presented at the Gender, Technology and Ethics Conference, Lulea, Sweden.

Kirejczyk, M. and van der Ploeg, I. (1992) 'Pregnant couples: medical technology and social constructions around fertility and reproduction', *Issues in Reproductive and Genetic Engineering* 5 (2): 113–25.

Kleinman, Arthur (1988) *The Illness Narratives: Suffering, Healing and the Human Condition*, New York: Basic Books.

Kolder, V., Gallagher, J. and Parsons, M. (1987) 'Court-ordered obstetrical intervention', *New England Journal of Medicine* 316: 1192–6.

Kuhn, Thomas (1970) *The Structure of Scientific Revolutions*, Chicago: University of Chicago Press.

Lacan, Jacques (1977a) 'The agency of the letter in the unconscious', in *Ecrits*, trans. A. Sheridan, London: Tavistock.

——(1977b) 'The mirror stage as formative of the function of the I' in *Ecrits*, trans. A. Sheridan, London: Tavistock.

Laqueur, Thomas (1990a) *Making Sex: Body and Gender from the Greeks to Freud*, Cambridge, MA: Harvard University Press.

——(1990b) 'The facts of fatherhood', in Marianne Hirsch and Evelyn Fox Keller (eds) *Conflicts in Feminism*, London: Routledge.

Leder, Drew (1984) 'Medicine and paradigms of embodiment', *Journal of Medicine and Philosophy* 9: 29–43.

——(1990) *The Absent Body*, Chicago: University of Chicago Press.

Lloyd, G.E.R. (1966) *Polarity and Analogy: Two Types of Argumentation in Early Greek Thought*, Cambridge: Cambridge University Press.

Lloyd, Genevieve (1984) *The Man of Reason: 'Male' and 'Female' in Western Philosophy*, London: Methuen.

——(1989) 'The Man of Reason' in Anne Garry and Marilyn Pearsall (eds) *Women, Knowledge and Reality*, London: Unwin Hyman.

Lochrie, K. (1991) *Margery Kempe and Translations of the Flesh*, Baltimore, PA: University of Pennsylvania Press.

Locke, John (1975) *An Essay Concerning Human Understanding*, ed. P.H. Nidditch, Oxford: Clarendon Press.

Lorber, Judith (1989) 'Choice, gift, or patriarchal bargain? Women's consent to *in vitro* fertilisation in male infertility', *Hypatia* 4 (3): 23–36.

Lorde, Audre (1984) 'Age, race, class and sex: women redefining difference', in *Sister/Outsider*, Trumansburg: Crossing Press.

Lorraine, Tamsin (1990) *Gender, Identity and the Production of Meaning*, Boulder, CO: Westview Press.

Lupton, Deborah (1994) *Medicine as Culture: Illness, Disease and the Body in Western Societies*, London: Sage.

——(1995) *The Imperative of Health*, London: Sage.

Lyotard, Jean-François (1984) *The Postmodern Condition: a Report on Knowledge*, Manchester: Manchester University Press.

McGuire, Maureen and Alexander, Nancy (1985) 'Artificial insemination of single women', *Fertility and Sterility* 43 (2): 182–4.

MacIntyre, Alasdair (1984) 'Does applied ethics rest on a mistake?' *The Monist* 67: 498–513.

Maclean, Anne (1993) *The Elimination of Morality: Reflections on Utilitarianism and Bioethics*, London: Routledge.

Maclean, Ian (1980) *The Renaissance Notion of Woman: a Study in the Fortunes of Scholasticism and Medical Science in European Intellectual Life*, Cambridge: Cambridge University Press.

McMinn, R.M.H. (1990) *Last's Anatomy: Regional and Applied*, 38th edn, Edinburgh: Churchill Livingstone.

McNay, Lois (1992) *Foucault and Feminism: Power, Gender and the Self*, Cambridge: Polity Press.

Manning, Rita (1992) 'Just caring', in Eve Browning Cole and Susan Coultrap-McQuin (eds) *Explorations in Feminist Ethics*, Bloomington: Indiana University Press.

Martin, Biddy and Mohanty, Chandra Talpade (1988) 'Feminist politics: what's home got to do with it?' in Teresa de Lauretis (ed.) *Feminist Studies/Critical Studies*, London: Macmillan.

Martin, Emily (1991) 'The egg and the sperm: how science has constructed a romance based on stereotypical male-female roles', *Signs* 16 (3): 485–501.

Martin, J., Meltzer, H. and Elliot, D. (1988) *The Prevalence of Disability among Adults*, London: HMSO.

May, Carl (1993) 'Reflexivity, self-identity, and self-help', *Occasional Papers* No. 3, Department of General Practice, University of Liverpool.

Medical Notes in Parliament (1943) 'Artificial insemination', in *British Medical Journal* 14 Aug.: 219.

Merleau-Ponty, Maurice (1962) *Phenomenology of Perception*, London: Routledge & Kegan Paul.

Mitchell, Juliet and Rose, Jacqueline (eds) (1982) *Feminine Sexuality: Jacques Lacan and the Ecole Freudienne*, London: Macmillan Press.

Moi, Toril (1985) *Sexual/Textual Politics*, London: Methuen.

Morgan, Kathryn Pauly (1988) 'Women and moral madness', in Lorraine Code, Sheila Mullett and Christine Overall (eds) *Feminist Perspectives: Philosophical Essays on Method and Morals*, Toronto: University of Toronto Press.

——(1989) 'Of woman born? How old-fashioned! New reproductive technologies and women's oppression', in Christine Overall (ed.) *The Future of Human Reproduction*, Toronto: The Women's Press.

Moulton, Janice (1989) 'The myth of the neutral man' in Ann Garry and Marilyn Pearsall (eds) *Women, Knowledge and Reality*, London: Unwin Hyman.

Mundinus (1541) *Anatomia*, Marburg: Johannes Dryander.

Natanson v *Kline* (1960) 186 Kan 393.

Nettleton, Sarah (1995) *The Sociology of Health and Illness*, London: Polity Press.

Neuberg, R. (1992) *So You Want to Have a Baby*, Serono Laboratories UK Ltd.

Nicholson, Linda J. (ed.) (1990) *Feminism/Postmodernism*, London: Routledge.

Noddings, Nel (1984) *Caring: a Feminine Approach to Ethics and Moral Education*, Berkeley: University of California Press.

Nye, Andrea (1989) *Feminist Theories and the Philosophies of Man*, London: Routledge.

Oakley, Ann (1980) *Women Confined*, Oxford: Martin Robertson.

O'Brien, Mary (1981) *The Politics of Reproduction*, London: Routledge & Kegan Paul.

OPCS (1994) *General Household Survey, 1992*, London: HMSO.

Orbach, Susie (1979) *Fat is a Feminist Issue*, London: Hamlyn.

Overall, Christine (1987) *Ethics and Human Reproduction: a Feminist Analysis*, London: Allen & Unwin.

—— (ed.) (1989) *The Future of Human Reproduction*, Toronto: The Women's Press.

Paton, H.J. (1961) *The Moral Law: Kant's 'Groundwork of the Metaphysic of Morals'*, London: Hutchinson University Library.

Pearsall, Marilyn (ed.) (1986) *Women and Values*, Belmont, CA: Wadsworth.

Pellegrino, Edmund D. and Thomasma, David C. (1988) *For the Patient's Good*, Oxford: Oxford University Press.

Pellikaan-Engel, Maja (ed.) (1992) *Against Patriarchal Thinking*, Amsterdam: VU University Press.

Petchesky, Rosalind P. (1987) 'Foetal images: the power of visual culture in the politics of reproduction' in Michelle Stanworth (ed.) *Reproductive Technologies: Gender, Motherhood and Medicine*, Cambridge: Polity Press.

Philips, E.D. (1987) *Aspects of Greek Medicine*, Philadelphia: The Charles Press.

Plato (1965) *Timaeus*, trans. H.P. Lee, Harmondsworth: Penguin.

Porter, Elisabeth (1991) *Women and Moral Identity*, London: Allen & Unwin.

Porter, M. (1990) 'Professional–client relationships', in S. Cunningham-Burley and N. McKeganey (eds) *Readings in Medical Sociology*, London: Routledge.

Price, Janet and Shildrick, Margrit (1995) 'Mapping the colonial body: sexual economies and the state in colonial India', in T.P. Foley, L. Pilkington, S. Ryder and E. Tilley (eds) *Gender and Colonialism*, Galway: Galway University Press.

R v *Ethical Committee of St Mary's Hospital (Manchester), ex parte H* (1988) 1 FLR 512.

Rawlinson, Mary C. (1987) 'Foucault's strategy: knowledge, power and the specificity of truth', *Journal of Medicine and Philosophy* 12 (4): 371–97.

Rawls, John (1972) *A Theory of Justice*, Oxford: Oxford University Press.

Raymond, Janice (1987) 'Fetalists and feminists', in Patricia Spallone and Deborah Lynn Steinberg (eds) *Made to Order: the Myth of Reproductive and Genetic Progress*, Oxford: Pergamon Press.

——(1990) 'Of ice and men: the big chill over women's reproductive rights', *Issues in Reproductive and Genetic Engineering* 3 (1): 45–50.

Re S, Adult: Refusal of Treatment (1992) 4 All ER 671.

Riley, Denise (1988) *'Am I That Name?' Feminism and the Category of 'Women' in History*, London: Macmillan.

Rogers, Sandra (1989) 'Pregnancy as justification for loss of juridical autonomy' in Christine Overall (ed.) *The Future of Human Reproduction*, Toronto: The Women's Press.

Rousseau, Jean-Jacques (1984) *Of the Social Contract and Discourse on Political Economy*, trans. C.M. Sherover, New York: Harper & Row.

Royal College of General Practitioners (1987) *The Front Line of the Health Service: College Response to Primary Health Care*, London: RCGP.

Ruddick, Sara (1990a) *Maternal Thinking: Towards a Politics of Peace*, London: Women's Press.

——(1990b) 'Thinking about fathers' in Marianne Hirsch and Evelyn Fox Keller (eds) *Conflicts in Feminism*, London: Routledge.

Sartre, Jean-Paul (1958) *Being and Nothingness: an Essay on Phenomenological Ontology*, London: Methuen.

Saunders, J.B. de C.M. and O'Malley, C.D. (1950) *The Illustrations from the Works of Andreas Vesalius*, Cleveland: World Publishing Co.

Saussure, Ferdinand de (1960) *Course in General Linguistics*, London: Peter Owen.

Sawicki, Jana (1991) *Disciplining Foucault: Feminism, Power and the Body*, London: Routledge.

Sayers, Janet (1986) *Sexual Contradictions: Psychology, Psychoanalysis, and Feminism*, London: Tavistock Publications.

Schenck, David (1986) 'The texture of embodiment: foundation for medical ethics', *Human Studies* 9: 43–54.

Schloendorff v *Society of New York Hospital* (1914) 105 NE 92.

Schopenhauer, Arthur (1965) *On the Basis of Morality*, trans. E.F.J. Payne, Indianapolis: Bobbs-Merrill.

Schor, Naomi (1989) 'Dreaming dissymmetry: Barthes, Foucault and sexual difference' in Elizabeth Weed (ed.) *Coming to Terms: Feminism, Theory, Politics*, London: Routledge.

Scutt, Jocelynne A. (ed.) (1990) *The Baby Machine: Reproductive Technology and the Commercialisation of Motherhood*, London: Merlin Press.

Seedhouse, David (1986) *Health: the Foundations for Achievement*, Chichester: John Wiley.

——(1988) *Ethics: the Heart of Health Care*, Chichester: John Wiley.

Sherwin, Susan (1992) *No Longer Patient: Feminist Ethics and Health Care*, Philadelphia: Temple University Press.

Shildrick, Margrit (1992) 'Women, bodies and consent', in Maja Pellikaan-Engel (ed.) *Against Patriarchal Thinking*, Amsterdam: VU University Press.

——(1997) 'Mis(sed) conceptions: NRTs and ontological anxiety', *Journal of Medicine and Philosophy* 22.

Shildrick, Margrit and Price, Janet (1994) 'Splitting the difference: adventures in the anatomy and embodiment of women', in Gabriele Griffin Marianne Hester, Shirin Rai and Sasha Roseneil (eds) *Stirring It: Challenges for Feminism*, London: Taylor & Francis.

Sidaway v *Board of Governors of the Bethlem Royal and the Maudsley Hospital* (1985) 1 All ER 643.

Siegemund, Justine (1723) *Die konigl. preussische und churbrandenb*, Berlin: J.A Rüdiger.

Singer, Linda (1993) *Erotic Welfare: Sexual Theory and Politics in the Age of Epidemic*, London: Routledge.

Singer, Peter (ed.) (1986) *Applied Ethics*, Oxford: Oxford University Press.

Singer, Peter and Wells, Deane (1983) '*In vitro* fertilisation: the major issues', *Journal of Medical Ethics* 9 (4): 192–9.

Smart, Carol (1989) 'Power and the politics of child custody', in Carol Smart and Selma Sevenhuijsen (eds) *Child Custody and the Politics of Gender*, London: Routledge.

Smith-Rosenberg, Carroll (1984) 'The hysterical woman: sex roles and role conflict in nineteenth-century America', in N Black, D. Boswell, A. Gray, S. Murphy and J. Popay (eds) *Health and Disease*, Milton Keynes: Open University Press.

Spallone, Patricia (1989) *Beyond Conception: the New Politics of Reproduction*, London: Macmillan.

Spallone, Patricia and Steinberg, Deborah Lynn (eds) (1987) *Made to Order: the Myth of Reproductive and Genetic Progress*, Oxford: Pergamon Press.

Spelman, Elizabeth V. (1990) *Inessential Woman: Problems of Exclusion in Feminist Thought*, London: Women's Press.

Spitzack, Carole (1987) 'Confession and signification: the systematic inscription of body consciousness', *Journal of Medicine and Philosophy* 12 (4): 357–71.

Spivak, Gayatri Chakravorty (1987) 'Displacement and the discourse of woman', in Mark Krupnick (ed.) *Displacement: Derrida and After*, Bloomington: Indiana University Press.

——(1988) *In Other Worlds: Essays in Cultural Politics*, London: Routledge.

——(1989a) 'Feminism and deconstruction, again: negotiating with unacknowledged masculinism', in Teresa Brennan (ed.) *Between Feminism and Psychoanalysis*, London: Routledge.

——(1989b) 'In a word', interview with Ellen Rooney, *differences* 1 (2): 124–56.

——(1990) *The Post-colonial Critic: Interviews, Strategies, Dialogues*, ed. Sarah Harasym, London: Routledge.

——(1992) 'French feminism revisited: ethics and politics', in Judith Butler and Joan W. Scott (eds) *Feminists Theorize the Political*, London: Routledge.

Stanworth, Michelle (ed.) (1987) *Reproductive Technologies: Gender, Motherhood and Medicine*, Cambridge: Polity Press.

——(1990) 'Birth pangs: conceptive technologies and the threat to motherhood', in Marianne Hirsch and Evelyn Fox Keller (eds) *Conflicts in Feminism*, London: Routledge.

Strathern, Marilyn (1992) *Reproducing the Future: Essays on Anthropology, Kinship and the New Reproductive Technologies*, New York: Routledge.

Swartz, Martha (1992) 'Pregnant woman vs. fetus: a dilemma for hospital ethics committees', *Cambridge Quarterly of Healthcare Ethics* 1 (1): 51–63.

Thomasma, David C. (1992) 'Models of the doctor–patient relationship and the ethics committee: Part One', *Cambridge Quarterly of Healthcare Ethics* 1 (1): 11–31.

Thompson, Janna (1983) 'Women and the high priests of reason', *Radical Philosophy* 34: 10–14.

Tuana, Nancy (1988) 'The weaker seed: the sexist bias of reproductive theory', *Hypatia* 3 (1): 35–59.

——(1992) 'Reading philosophy as a woman' in Maja Pellikaan-Engel (ed.) *Against Patriarchal Thinking*, Amsterdam: VU University Press.

——(1993) *The Less Noble Sex: Scientific, Religious, and Philosophical Conceptions of Women's Nature*, Bloomington: Indiana University Press.

Turner, Bryan S. (1987) *Medical Power and Social Knowledge*, London: Sage Publications.

——(1992) *Regulating Bodies: Essays in Medical Sociology*, London: Routledge.

Valverde de Hamusco, Juan (1560) *Anatomia del corpo humano*, Rome: A. Salamanca.

Vesalius, Andreas (1543) *De humani corporis fabrica*, Basel: J. Operinus.

Warnock, Mary (ed.) (1979) *Utilitarianism; On Liberty; and Essay on Bentham*, Glasgow: Collins.

——(1985) 'The artificial family', in Michael Lockwood (ed.) *Moral Dilemmas in Modern Medicine*, Oxford: Oxford University Press.

Warnock Report (1984) *Report of the Committee of Inquiry into Human Fertilisation and Embryology*, Cmnd 9314, London: HMSO.

Weed, Elizabeth (ed.) (1989) *Coming to Terms: Feminism, Theory, Politics*, London: Routledge.

Weedon, Chris (1987) *Feminist Practice and Poststructuralist Theory*, Oxford: Blackwell.

Wendell, Susan (1992) 'Toward a feminist theory of disability', in Helen Bequaert Holmes and Laura M. Purdy (eds) *Feminist Perspectives in Medical Ethics*, Bloomington: Indiana University Press.

Whitbeck, Caroline (1989) 'A different reality: feminist ontology' in A. Garry and M. Pearsall (eds) *Women, Knowledge and Reality*, London: Unwin Hyman.

Whitford, Margaret (1991) *Luce Irigaray: Philosophy in the Feminine*, London: Routledge.

Williams, A. (1994) 'Economics, society and health care ethics', in R. Gillon (ed.) *Principles of Health Care Ethics*, Chichester: John Wiley.

Williams, B. (1985) *Ethics and the Limits of Philosophy*, London: Fontana.

Williams, P.L. (ed.) (1995) *Gray's Anatomy* 38th edn, Edinburgh: Churchill Livingstone.

Young, Iris Marion (1984) 'Pregnant embodiment: subjectivity and alienation', *Journal of Medicine and Philosophy* 9: 45–62.

——(1990) *Throwing Like a Girl and Other Essays in Feminist Philosophy and Social Theory*, Bloomington: Indiana University Press.

Ziebland, Sue, Fitzpatrick, Ray and Jenkinson, Crispin (1993) 'Tacit models of disability underlying health status instruments', *Social Science and Medicine* 37 (1): 69–77.

Glossary of abbreviations

AI   Artificial insemination. A simple procedure by which spermatozoa are deposited in a woman's vagina other than by sexual intercourse.

AID   Artificial insemination by donor. Sperm from donors are used to circumvent the sterility of the male partner.

AR   Assisted reproduction. The preferred term for all the procedures by which fertilisation is achieved other than by sexual intercourse between the primary couple.

BPAS   British Pregnancy Advisory Service. A non-profit-making charitable organisation which at one time offered infertility services, mainly AI, to women unable to obtain help through the NHS.

DI   Donor insemination. (Replaces AID in current literature.)

DLA   Disability Living Allowance. A state benefit paid to claimants with long-term disabilities to enable them to purchase care, or items to alleviate their difficulties.

DNA   Deoxyribonucleic acid. The base material of human genes.

FINRRAGE Feminist International Network of Resistance to Reproductive and Genetic Engineering. (See also Chapter 6, note 10.)

GIFT   Gamete intrafallopian transfer. A variant procedure of IVF by which collected sperm and ova are injected into a woman's fallopian tubes for fertilisation there.

HFEA   Human Fertilisation and Embryology Authority. The governmental body set up to oversee the implementation of the HFE Act, 1990.

HIV   Human Immunodeficiency Virus.

IRAGE   *Issues in Reproductive and Genetic Engineering, Journal of International Feminist Analysis.*

IVF   *In vitro* fertilisation. The process of achieving fertilisation outside the womb by mixing sperm and ova together in a glass Petri dish, prior to re-implantation. The source of the misnomer 'test-tube' baby.

NHS	National Health Service.
NRT	New reproductive technologies.
OPCS	Office of Population Censuses and Surveys. British government body handling demographic data.

Index

Page numbers indicated in **bold** refer to illustrations.